Resilient Communities: Navigating Public Health Challenges in Developing Nations

Authored by

Jalal-Eddeen Abubakar Saleh
Field Presence Cluster
World Health Organization, Nigeria

Resilient Communities: Navigating Public Health Challenges in Developing Nations

Author: Jalal-Eddeen Abubakar Saleh

ISBN (Online): 978-981-5305-60-9

ISBN (Print): 978-981-5305-61-6

ISBN (Paperback): 978-981-5305-62-3

Published by Bentham Science Publishers Pte. Ltd. Singapore. All Rights Reserved.

First published in 2025.

need for a court order if at any point you breach any terms of this License Agreement. In no event will any delay or failure by Bentham Science Publishers in enforcing your compliance with this License Agreement constitute a waiver of any of its rights.

3. You acknowledge that you have read this License Agreement, and agree to be bound by its terms and conditions. To the extent that any other terms and conditions presented on any website of Bentham Science Publishers conflict with, or are inconsistent with, the terms and conditions set out in this License Agreement, you acknowledge that the terms and conditions set out in this License Agreement shall prevail.

Bentham Science Publishers Pte. Ltd.
80 Robinson Road #02-00
Singapore 068898
Singapore
Email: subscriptions@benthamscience.net

BENTHAM SCIENCE

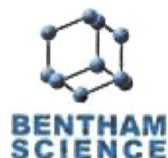

CONTENTS

FOREWORD

In a world that grapples with diverse challenges, there is a beacon of hope that shines brightly – the resilience of communities. The indomitable spirit of these communities, especially in the face of public health challenges in developing nations, is a testament to the power of human determination and solidarity. It is with great honor and enthusiasm that I introduce this book, "Resilient Communities: Navigating Public Health Challenges in Developing Nations", a profound and timely exploration of the intrinsic transformative potential within us.

As a long-time advocate of global health equity, I have had the privilege of having firsthand experienced the remarkable impact of the resilience of communities in shaping public health outcomes. This book serves as an illuminating guide to navigating the complexities and opportunities that are present in the pursuit of health and well-being for all.

The chapters provide an insight into the salient public health challenges in developing nations. The author skilfully navigates the intricate interplay of socio-economic factors, health disparities, and cultural diversity that shape the health landscape. Importantly, he underscores the need to approach these challenges with empathy, recognizing that resilient communities emerge not merely from strength but from compassionate collaboration.

The principle and the power of community-based participatory approaches form the basis of the book. Empowering communities to become architects of their health destiny is not only visionary but an imperative step towards sustainable progress. The author delves into the significance of community engagement, where the voices of those affected by health challenges take center stage in shaping interventions and strategies that resonate with their unique contexts.

In traversing the realms of communicable and non-communicable diseases, maternal and child health, and essential water, sanitation, and hygiene interventions, the book highlights the importance of holistic health solutions. It celebrates the role of preventive measures and early interventions, acknowledging that resilient communities thrive when equipped with the tools to proactively safeguard their well-being.

Moreover, the emphasis on healthcare infrastructure and access is pivotal in understanding the dynamics of public health implementation. With inspiring case studies, the book showcases how innovation, technology, and community-driven initiatives can bridge gaps in healthcare delivery, especially in resource-constrained settings.

While public health challenges may be daunting, the book illuminates the path of resilience amidst adversity. It addresses the vital role of mental health and psychosocial support in nurturing well-being and emphasizes the significance of disaster preparedness and community resilience in safeguarding lives during crises.

In a transformative and empowering chapter, the book highlights the indispensable role of the female gender in driving positive change in public health. It promotes gender equity and provides opportunities for women and girls to lead, creating a powerful force that propels communities toward better health outcomes.

The book resonates with the spirit of innovation, revealing the vast potential of technology in healthcare, from revolutionary mobile health initiatives to data-driven solutions that empower decision-making and enhance impact.

Ultimately, "Resilient Communities" transcends theory and offers a compelling call to action. By recognizing that health systems and governance are the bedrock of sustainable progress, the book encourages collaboration and commitment to building a brighter health future for developing nations.

To the author who has showcased his expertise, passion, and dedication in this book, I extend my commendation. Your painstaking efforts have produced useful guidance for policymakers, public health professionals, community leaders, and advocates.

To all readers who embark on this transformative journey, I invite you to draw inspiration from the stories shared within these pages. May you be moved to embrace the resilience within your communities, ignite change, and champion the cause of health and well-being for all.

Together, let us honor the strength of resilient communities and collectively navigate the path towards a healthier and more equitable world.

Babatunji Abayomi Omotara
University of Maiduguri
Maiduguri 600104, Borno
Nigeria

PREFACE

In the diverse tapestry of our world, some communities inspire hope and admiration with their unwavering spirit and ability to rise above adversity. These are the resilient communities – bastions of strength in the face of daunting public health challenges. As I turn my attention to developing nations, I find myself immersed in a dynamic landscape where the pursuit of health equity knows no bounds.

This book, "Resilient Communities: Navigating Public Health Challenges in Developing Nations", explores the remarkable power that lies within communities to transform their health outcomes. It is a journey through the complexities of public health in resource-constrained settings, guided by the unwavering belief in the potential of collective action and community empowerment.

I have witnessed the fortitude of these communities, and this book is a testament to their indomitable spirit. It is also a tribute to the tireless efforts of public health professionals, policymakers, community leaders, and advocates who work tirelessly to bring about positive change.

In the opening chapters, I set the stage, delving into the intricacies of public health in developing nations. I unravel the web of factors that influence health outcomes, from socioeconomic disparities to prevailing diseases, and emphasize the importance of addressing health inequities with a lens of compassion and understanding.

The heart of this book lies in its exploration of community resilience and the transformative impact of community engagement. I highlight the power of a community-based participatory approach, where people affected by health challenges become change agents, shaping interventions that best suit their needs and context.

Throughout the chapters, I traverse the terrain of communicable diseases, non-communicable diseases, maternal and child health, and the critical importance of water, sanitation, and hygiene interventions. I explored the intricate relationship between nutrition and health and the vital role of mental health and psychosocial support in resilient communities.

Healthcare infrastructure and access form an integral part of the journey. I discussed innovative solutions leveraging technology to bridge healthcare delivery gaps and empower communities to lead healthier lives.

As I delved into the realm of disaster preparedness and resilience, I acknowledged the need for a proactive approach to safeguarding communities from the impact of natural disasters and emergencies.

Given that women and girls emerge as influential change-makers in public health, I underscored the importance of gender equity and the empowerment of women and girls, recognizing their indispensable role in building healthier societies.

Throughout the pages of this book, I celebrated the triumphs of technology and innovation in public health. From mobile health initiatives to digital data collection and analysis tools, I witnessed how technology can revolutionize healthcare access and delivery.

Amidst all these efforts, I delved into the essence of health systems and governance. I explored the significance of solid leadership, capacity building, and sustainable development to lay a foundation for lasting health resilience.

As I approached the final chapters, I glimpsed the vision of resilient health futures for developing nations. I integrated public health into sustainable development goals, envisioning a world where every community thrives and everyone is empowered to lead a healthier, more fulfilling life. I explored the critical issues surrounding weak routine immunization, poor leadership and governance, poor coordination of disease outbreaks and response, and non-performing primary healthcare centers.

In the book, the reader would find enlightening case studies strategically placed after the various chapters. These case studies utilize fictional settings to vividly exemplify how innovation, technology, and community-driven initiatives come together to address healthcare delivery gaps, especially in locations with limited resources. Ultimately, this book is more than a compilation of knowledge; it is an invitation to action. It is a call to embrace the resilience within us all and recognize that the most potent solutions emerge when we work together as a global community united in purpose and compassion.

To every reader who embarks on this journey, may the stories within these pages ignite your imagination and inspire your commitment to advancing public health in developing nations. Together, we champion resilient communities and pave the way for a healthier, more equitable world.

Disclaimer:

The views expressed in this book are mine and do not reflect the official position or policies of the WHO. Similarly, the content of this book ensured objectivity, avoided being impartial, and was not influenced by my affiliation with the WHO.

Jalal-Eddeen Abubakar Saleh
Field Presence Cluster
World Health Organization, Nigeria

DEDICATION

To the resilient communities worldwide, whose unwavering spirit and strength illuminate the path towards better health and inspire us to navigate challenges with courage and compassion.

To the public health professionals, policymakers, and advocates whose tireless dedication and unwavering commitment bring hope and progress to communities in need, your passion drives positive change.

To the women and girls, the catalysts of transformation and empowerment, whose vision and leadership shape healthier futures, your impact knows no bounds.

To future generations whose well-being is our collective responsibility, may this book be a guiding light towards a world where health and equity flourish for all.

CHAPTER 1

Introduction

Abstract: This chapter introduces the concept of resilient communities as vital players in addressing public health challenges, particularly in developing nations. It emphasises the significance of community engagement and empowerment in navigating complex health obstacles. The overview of public health challenges in these nations underscores the need for innovative, community-driven solutions. Through case studies and real-world examples, the chapter sets the stage for understanding the transformative potential of resilient communities in shaping healthier societies.

Keywords: Community engagement, Community empowerment, Developing nations, Public health challenges, Resilient communities.

INTRODUCTION

Resilient communities stand as pillars of strength amidst daunting public health challenges in developing nations. Their proactive approach, rooted in collective action and innovation, enables them to not only withstand adversity but also drive positive change. By leveraging local knowledge and resources, they emerge as architects of their health destinies, fostering inclusive and sustainable health solutions.

Developing nations face a myriad of public health challenges, from infectious diseases and non-communicable diseases to maternal and child health disparities and inadequate healthcare infrastructure. Despite these obstacles, there is growing momentum towards collaborative solutions that prioritise health equity and community empowerment. This section explores the interconnected factors contributing to health disparities and the transformative initiatives aimed at building healthier societies.

Community engagement and empowerment are fundamental to addressing public health challenges effectively. By involving communities in decision-making processes and nurturing their agency, public health interventions become more contextually relevant and sustainable. Through meaningful engagement, communities emerge as catalysts for change, driving initiatives that promote health equity and resilience at the grassroots level.

The Significance of Resilient Communities in Addressing Public Health Challenges

In the ever-changing landscape of global health, few forces rival the transformative power of resilient communities. These dynamic entities, often found in the heart of developing nations, are uniquely able to navigate and address daunting public health challenges with unwavering determination. Their significance lies in their capacity to withstand adversity and their remarkable ability to bounce back, adapt, and grow more robust in the face of daunting health obstacles [1, 2].

At the heart of the concept of resilience lies the essence of human fortitude and solidarity. Resilient communities exhibit a remarkable sense of cohesion, unity, and collective spirit that binds individuals together to pursue health and well-being. They are not passive bystanders waiting for external solutions but actively engage in co-creating and implementing interventions that respond to their specific needs and context. In doing so, they become architects of their health destinies, playing a pivotal role in shaping the trajectory of public health in their regions [1, 2].

Resilient communities emerge as a critical lifeline in developing nations, where resources may be scarce, infrastructure limited, and access to healthcare challenging. They epitomize the power of human resilience, leveraging their local knowledge, cultural wisdom, and social capital to navigate complex health challenges. Their inherent strengths extend far beyond their ability to withstand shocks; they actively seek opportunities to mobilize resources, advocate for their rights, and forge partnerships with various stakeholders, including public health professionals, policymakers, non-governmental organizations, and international agencies [1, 2].

Resilient communities are exemplars of adaptability, creativity, and innovation. Faced with ever-evolving health threats, they demonstrate a remarkable capacity to improvise and find solutions that resonate with their cultural norms and beliefs. This resourcefulness is often borne out of necessity, as they transform constraints into opportunities for growth and progress. Their ability to leverage technology, traditional knowledge, and community-based practices empowers them to build sustainable public health responses that stand the test of time [1, 2].

One of the most compelling aspects of resilient communities is their commitment to leaving no one behind. Inclusive and equitable, they place a premium on ensuring that the most vulnerable and marginalized members of society are not overlooked in health interventions. Their focus on collective well-being extends beyond individual health; it encompasses the social, economic, and environmental determinants that shape community health outcomes. Addressing these underlying factors fortifies the foundation upon which resilient communities thrive [1, 2].

Resilient communities are catalysts for change, inspiring hope and progress despite insurmountable challenges. Their success stories illuminate the transformative potential of local-level action and community-driven initiatives. These stories remind us that while the road to better health may be arduous, it is paved with hope, determination, and resilience [1, 2].

In this book, "Resilient Communities: Navigating Public Health Challenges in Developing Nations", the journey will explore the multifaceted significance of resilient communities in addressing public health challenges. The book will delve into their unique characteristics, the contextual factors that shape a community's resilience, and the strategies they employ to drive positive change. Through the lens of resilience, it will seek to understand how communities can become active participants in shaping public health outcomes and how their resilience can be harnessed to build sustainable, inclusive, and equitable health solutions [1 - 3]. (Figs. **1** and **2**) vividly contrast the socio-economic landscapes, illustrating a typical rural sub-Saharan African community in Fig. (**1**) and a mid-income country community in Fig. (**2**), highlighting the diverse contexts within which public health challenges are navigated.

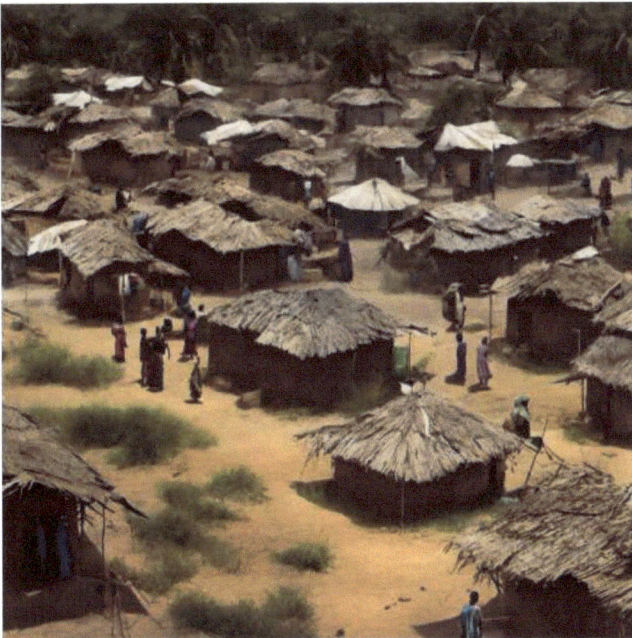

Fig. (1). A community in a typical rural sub-Saharan African setting.

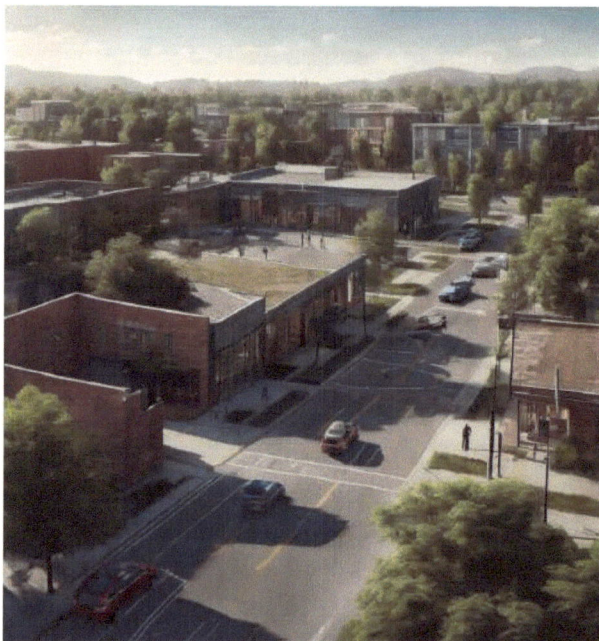

Fig. (2). A community in a mid-income country.

This section examines the power of collective action, community empowerment, and innovation through case studies, evidence-based practices, and real-world examples. It recognizes that resilient communities are not passive recipients of external aid; instead, they are change-makers, leaders, and trailblazers in the pursuit of healthier, more resilient societies [1 - 4].

As we traverse the chapters of this book, the reader will discover the essence of resilience and its profound impact on public health in developing nations. Together, we will uncover the inherent strengths within communities and chart a course towards a brighter and healthier future for all [1 - 5].

Overview of Public Health Challenges in Developing Nations

In the vast expanse of our world, public health is an ever-evolving landscape shaped by myriad factors that define populations' health and well-being. Nowhere are these challenges more pronounced than in developing nations, where complex and interconnected issues converge to create unique health disparities and obstacles. This introductory chapter offers an overview of these nations' multifaceted public health challenges, shedding light on the pressing issues that demand urgent attention, collective action, and innovative solutions [6].

A complex interplay of socio-economic factors is at the heart of the public health challenges in developing nations. Poverty, lack of access to education, inadequate sanitation, and limited healthcare infrastructure create a web of interlocking challenges that impede health progress. These factors perpetuate a cycle of poor health outcomes, particularly in vulnerable and marginalized communities, leading to increased morbidity and mortality rates [6, 7].

Infectious diseases remain a formidable adversary in the developing world. From malaria and tuberculosis to HIV/AIDS and neglected tropical diseases, these communicable diseases continue to exert a heavy toll on human lives and economies. The burden is exacerbated by factors such as inadequate healthcare resources, fragmented healthcare systems, and challenges in disease surveillance and control [6, 7].

Amidst the ongoing battle against communicable diseases, non-communicable diseases (NCDs) are rapidly emerging as a major public health concern. The rising prevalence of conditions like cardiovascular diseases, diabetes, cancer, and respiratory illnesses presents a dual burden for healthcare systems already grappling with infectious diseases. The transition towards unhealthy lifestyles, including poor nutrition, sedentary behaviour, and tobacco use, further amplifies the impact of NCDs in developing countries [6, 7].

Maternal and child health is a critical area where the health disparities are particularly acute. High maternal mortality rates, inadequate access to prenatal care, and limited access to skilled birth attendants contribute to the vulnerability of expectant mothers and newborns. Malnutrition and preventable childhood illnesses continue to affect child's health, compromising their growth and development [6, 7].

Access to safe drinking water, proper sanitation, and hygiene practices is an ongoing challenge in many developing nations. Lack of access to clean water sources, inadequate sanitation facilities, and poor hygiene practices contribute to the prevalence of waterborne diseases and undermine efforts to promote health and prevent infections.

Furthermore, mental health is an often overlooked and stigmatized aspect of public health in developing nations. Limited resources for mental health services, a lack of awareness, and cultural stigma surrounding mental illness contribute to inadequate care and support for individuals dealing with mental health challenges [6, 7].

Healthcare systems in developing nations face significant barriers, including limited funding, insufficient healthcare workforce, and infrastructural challenges.

The shortage of skilled healthcare professionals, especially in remote and underserved areas, exacerbates healthcare disparities and hampers timely access to essential medical services [6, 7].

While these public health challenges may seem daunting, developing nations are hubs of innovation, resilience, and community engagement. Governments, non-governmental organizations, international agencies, and communities are coming together to forge solutions that address these challenges with determination and ingenuity. Pursuing health equity is no longer an isolated endeavour; it is a collective journey to empower communities, strengthen healthcare systems, and promote inclusive public health initiatives [6, 7].

This book, "Resilient Communities: Navigating Public Health Challenges in Developing Nations", seeks to illuminate the complexities of these challenges, explore innovative strategies, and celebrate the progress made towards building healthier and more resilient societies. By examining real-world case studies, evidence-based practices, and transformative initiatives, we inspire readers to advocate for change, contributing to the transformative journey of global health equity for all [6, 7].

As the book embarks on this exploration, we should recognize that the path ahead may be arduous. However, we can create a healthier and more equitable world through understanding, collaboration, and compassion for generations to come [6, 7].

The Role of Community Engagement and Empowerment in Public Health

In the realm of public health, the role of communities extends far beyond being passive recipients of healthcare interventions; they are the heart and soul of transformative change. Community engagement and empowerment are essential pillars in pursuing effective and sustainable public health initiatives, especially in developing nations. This section of the introduction chapter explores the profound significance of community involvement, highlighting how their active participation can shape the trajectory of public health outcomes and drive positive, lasting impact [8, 9].

Community Engagement: A Catalyst for Change

At its core, community engagement embodies the principle of inclusivity and collaboration. It acknowledges the wisdom, experiences, and local knowledge within the community and recognizes the unique perspectives they bring to the table. By involving community members in every stage of the public health decision-making process - from planning and implementation to monitoring and evaluation - engagement ensures that interventions are culturally sensitive, contextually relevant, and responsive to the specific needs of the population.

Community engagement fosters ownership and accountability. When individuals actively participate in designing and implementing public health interventions, they develop a sense of responsibility towards the success and sustainability of those initiatives. This participatory approach enhances the likelihood of interventions being embraced and adopted by the community, as they are seen as products of collective efforts rather than externally imposed mandates [8, 9].

Empowerment: Nurturing Resilience and Agency

Empowerment is a transformative force that can uplift individuals and communities from a state of vulnerability to one of strength and agency. In public health, empowerment equips individuals with the knowledge, skills, and resources they need to make informed decisions about their health and well-being. It also fosters a sense of self-efficacy, instilling the belief that they have the power to influence positive health outcomes and lead healthier lives.

Empowered communities are likelier to take charge of their health and advocate for their rights. They become active partners in identifying health priorities, mobilizing resources, and collaborating with diverse stakeholders to address public health challenges. This sense of agency enables them to challenge systemic inequalities and advocate for equitable access to healthcare, social services, and resources essential for their well-being [8, 9].

Transforming Health at the Grassroots Level

The transformative potential of community engagement and empowerment lies in their ability to address the root causes of health disparities. By engaging communities in meaningful ways, public health interventions become contextually relevant and sustainable. This approach helps dismantle barriers that inhibit access to healthcare, such as cultural norms, gender inequalities, and socio-economic constraints.

At the grassroots level, community-driven initiatives have demonstrated remarkable success in tackling public health challenges. From community-based health workers providing essential care to local outreach programs promoting preventive health practices, these initiatives leverage the strengths and assets of the community to drive change. They showcase how public health can be transformed from a top-down approach to one firmly rooted in the unique needs and aspirations of the people it serves [8, 9].

Building Resilient Communities for a Healthier Future

In the context of public health challenges in developing nations, community engagement and empowerment are crucial to building resilient communities that can navigate adversities and thrive. The collaboration between communities, public health professionals, policymakers, and various stakeholders is a powerful force that can shape a healthier, more equitable future.

As we explore the transformative impact of community engagement and empowerment throughout this book, we celebrate the resilience, creativity, and agency of communities in driving positive change. By embracing these principles, we can co-create a path towards a world where public health initiatives are driven by the power of collective action and rooted in the core values of dignity, equity, and well-being for all [8, 9].

CONCLUSION

As we embark on this journey through the intricacies of public health in developing nations, it becomes evident that resilient communities are central to shaping healthier futures. By harnessing the power of community engagement, empowerment, and collective action, we can overcome seemingly insurmountable challenges and pave the way for a world where health is a fundamental human right and accessible to all.

REFERENCES

[1]   Patel SS, Rogers MB, Amlôt R, Rubin GJ. What Do We Mean by 'Community Resilience'? A Systematic Literature Review of How It Is Defined in the Literature. PLoS Curr 2017; 9: ecurrents.dis.db775aff25efc5ac4f0660ad9c9f7db2.

[2]   Biddle L, Wahedi K, Bozorgmehr K. Health system resilience: a literature review of empirical research. Health Policy Plan 2020; 35(8): 1084-109.
[http://dx.doi.org/10.1093/heapol/czaa032] [PMID: 32529253]

[3]   Chabrol F, David PM. How resilience affected public health research during COVID-19 and why we should abandon it. Glob Public Health 2023; 18(1): 2212750.
[http://dx.doi.org/10.1080/17441692.2023.2212750] [PMID: 37196668]

[4]   Wulff K, Donato D, Lurie N. What Is Health Resilience and How Can We Build It? Annu Rev Pub Health 2015; 36: 361-74.
[http://dx.doi.org/10.1146/annurev-publhealth-031914-122829]

[5]   Cutter SL, Barnes L, Berry M, et al. A place-based model for understanding community resilience to natural disasters. Glob Environ Change 2008; 18(4): 598-606.
[http://dx.doi.org/10.1016/j.gloenvcha.2008.07.013]

[6]   World Health Organization (2016). World Health Assembly, 69. Health in the 2030 Agenda for Sustainable Development. World Health Organization, 2016. Available from: https://apps.who.int/iris/handle/10665/252791

[7]   World Health Organization. Regional Office for Europe. Health systems respond to noncommunicable diseases: time for ambition: summary. World Health Organization. Regional Office for Europe, 2019.

Available from: https://apps.who.int/iris/handle/10665/329353

[8]   Rifkin SB. Examining the links between community participation and health outcomes: a review of the literature. Health Policy Plan 2014; 29(Suppl 2) (Suppl. 2): ii98-ii106.
[http://dx.doi.org/10.1093/heapol/czu076] [PMID: 25274645]

[9]   Wallerstein NB, Duran B. Using community-based participatory research to address health disparities. Health Promot Pract 2006; 7(3): 312-23.
[http://dx.doi.org/10.1177/1524839906289376] [PMID: 16760238]

CHAPTER 2

Understanding Public Health in Developing Nations

Abstract: This chapter delves into the intricate fabric of public health in developing nations, focusing on key health indicators, prevalent diseases, socioeconomic factors, health disparities, and inequities. Understanding these elements is crucial for crafting targeted interventions and fostering health equity. Through the exploration of case studies, this chapter illuminates the complex interplay of factors shaping public health outcomes in diverse communities.

Keywords: Developing nations, Health disparities, Health inequities, Key health indicators, Prevalent diseases, Public health, Socioeconomic factors.

INTRODUCTION

Understanding key health indicators and prevalent diseases is vital for assessing the health status of populations in developing nations. Life expectancy, maternal mortality ratio, under-five mortality rate, infant mortality rate, child malnutrition, and access to safe water and sanitation are critical indicators reflecting the overall well-being of communities. Prevalent diseases, including communicable diseases (CDs), non-communicable diseases (NCDs), and neglected tropical diseases (NTDs), pose significant health challenges and require targeted interventions to mitigate their impact.

Socioeconomic factors play a pivotal role in shaping public health outcomes in developing nations. Poverty, education, nutrition, limited access to healthcare, sanitation, and environmental conditions significantly impact health disparities. Addressing these determinants involves a range of comprehensive strategies, including but not limited to promoting economic development, enhancing education, improving healthcare access, ensuring food security, and mitigating environmental risks while also remaining open to other innovative and context-specific approaches. Health disparities and inequities pervade the public health landscape of developing nations, driven by social, economic, and cultural factors. Unequal access to healthcare services, maternal and child health disparities, infectious disease burden, NCD prevalence, and mental health challenges con-

Jalal-Eddeen Abubakar Saleh

tribute to disparities. Achieving health equity demands targeted interventions, policy reforms, and collaborative efforts to address the root causes of disparities and promote inclusive healthcare systems.

Key Health Indicators and Prevalent Diseases

In the complex tapestry of public health in developing nations, understanding key health indicators and prevalent diseases is essential to grasp the health status of populations and identify priority areas for intervention. Tables **2.1a** and **2.1b** show the key health indicators and prevalent diseases to guide the reader. These indicators serve as vital signposts, providing insights into the overall health and well-being of communities and the challenges they face. In this section, we will look into key health indicators and prevalent diseases that shape the public health landscape in developing nations [1, 2].

Table 2.1a. Key health indicators.

S. No.	Indicator	Remark
1.	Life Expectancy	Average number of years a person can expect to live; reflects the overall health and well-being of the population.
2.	Infant Mortality Rate	Number of deaths of infants under one year of age per 1,000 live births; indicates the quality of maternal and child healthcare.
3.	Maternal Mortality Rate	Number of maternal deaths per 100,000 live births; highlights the safety of pregnancy and childbirth.
4.	Under-5 Mortality Rate	Number of deaths of children under five years of age per 1,000 live births; reflects child health and access to healthcare.
5.	Malnutrition Rates	Rates of undernutrition (stunting, wasting) and overnutrition (obesity) among children and adults; indicates food security and dietary habits.
6.	Access to Clean Water & Sanitation	Percentage of the population with access to safe drinking water and proper sanitation facilities; critical for preventing waterborne diseases.
7.	Vaccination Coverage	Percentage of children and adults who receive essential vaccines; helps prevent infectious diseases.
8.	Prevalence of Infectious Diseases	Rates of diseases such as malaria, HIV/AIDS, tuberculosis, and neglected tropical diseases; is a significant health challenges in developing nations.
9.	Access to Healthcare Services	Availability and utilization of healthcare facilities, including hospitals, clinics, and primary care centers.
10.	Healthcare Worker Density	Number of healthcare professionals (doctors, nurses, midwives) per capita; reflects the availability of skilled healthcare providers.

(Table 2.1a) cont.....

S. No.	Indicator	Remark
11.	Health Expenditure	Total healthcare spending as a percentage of GDP; indicates the level of investment in the healthcare system.
12.	Health Insurance Coverage	Percentage of the population with access to health insurance or social protection schemes for healthcare.
13.	Epidemic Preparedness	The capacity of the healthcare system to respond to disease outbreaks, including surveillance, response plans, and healthcare infrastructure.
14.	Nutritional Programs	The presence and effectiveness of nutrition programs for vulnerable populations, such as pregnant women and children.
15.	Environmental Health	Measures of air and water pollution, access to safe cooking fuels, and exposure to environmental hazards.
16.	Education and Health Literacy	Levels of education and health literacy among the population, which influence health-seeking behaviors and understanding of healthcare information.
17.	Gender Disparities in Health	Gender-specific health indicators, including maternal health, reproductive health, and access to healthcare for women and girls.
18.	Mental Health Indicators	Rates of mental health conditions and access to mental healthcare services.
19.	Non-Communicable Diseases	Rates of non-communicable diseases (NCDs), such as diabetes, cardiovascular diseases, and cancer, which are becoming increasingly prevalent in developing nations.
20.	Social Determinants of Health	Factors such as income inequality, education, employment, and social support systems that impact overall health and well-being.

Table 2.1b. Prevalent diseases in developing nations.

S. No.	Disease	Remark
1.	Malaria	Mosquito-borne infectious disease, is a major health concern in many developing nations, particularly in sub-Saharan Africa, and can lead to severe illness and death if not treated promptly.
2.	HIV/AIDS	HIV/AIDS remains a significant health challenge, with many developing nations having high prevalence rates. Access to antiretroviral therapy and prevention programs is crucial.
3.	Tuberculosis (TB)	TB, an airborne bacterial infection, primarily affects the lungs. It is a major public health issue in many developing nations, and drug-resistant TB strains are a growing concern.
4.	Diarrhoeal Diseases	Diseases such as cholera, rotavirus, and E. coli infections can lead to severe diarrhea and dehydration, especially in areas with poor sanitation and limited access to clean water.

(Table 2.1b) cont.....

S. No.	Disease	Remark
5.	Respiratory Infections	Pneumonia and other respiratory infections remain common causes of illness and mortality in developing nations.
6.	NTDs	NTDs like schistosomiasis, lymphatic filariasis, and onchocerciasis disproportionately affect people, causing chronic health problems.
7.	Dengue Fever	Dengue, a mosquito-borne viral infection, can lead to severe flu-like symptoms and, in some cases, life-threatening complications. It is endemic in many tropical and subtropical regions.
8.	Chronic Diseases (NCDs)	NCDs like diabetes, cardiovascular diseases, and cancer are on the rise in developing nations due to changing lifestyles and diets.
9.	Malnutrition	Both undernutrition and overnutrition (obesity) can be prevalent in developing nations, leading to a range of health issues.
10.	Vector-Borne Diseases	Diseases transmitted by vectors, such as Zika virus, Chikungunya, and leishmaniasis, are of concern in many developing regions.
11.	Waterborne Diseases	Contaminated water sources can lead to waterborne diseases like typhoid, cholera, and dysentery.
12.	Parasitic Infections	Parasitic diseases like schistosomiasis, intestinal worms, and trypanosomiasis are endemic in some developing nations.
13.	Childhood Diseases	VPDs - measles, polio, and whooping cough can still pose threats to children's health in some areas with low vaccination coverage.
14.	Emerging Diseases	Emerging infectious diseases, such as Ebola and Zika virus outbreaks.
15.	Mental Health Conditions	These issues are increasingly recognized as important public health concerns due to limited mental healthcare services.
16.	Education and Health Literacy	Levels of education and health literacy among the population, which influence health-seeking behaviors and understanding of healthcare information.
17.	Gender Disparities in Health	Gender-specific health indicators, including maternal health, reproductive health, and access to healthcare for women and girls.
18.	Mental Health Indicators	Rates of mental health conditions and access to mental healthcare services.

Understanding the factors influencing public health in these regions is essential for crafting effective strategies and interventions. This section discusses a few of the Key Health Indicators.

Key Health Indicators

In the complex tapestry of global health, the significance of "Key Health Indicators" cannot be overstated. These indicators serve as the compass guiding public health policies, interventions, and initiatives in both developed and developing nations. They offer a lens through which we can understand the well-being of populations, assess healthcare systems, and work toward achieving health equity for all. Developing nations face unique challenges and opportunities on their journey toward improving the health and well-being of their populations.

Life Expectancy: Life expectancy at birth is a fundamental measure of a population's overall health and well-being. In developing nations, life expectancy often varies significantly, influenced by factors such as access to healthcare, nutrition, sanitation, and socio-economic disparities. High infant mortality rates can impact life expectancy, emphasizing the need for maternal and child health interventions.

Maternal Mortality Ratio: The maternal mortality ratio (MMR) is a critical indicator of maternal health, reflecting the number of maternal deaths per 100,000 live births. In developing nations, maternal mortality remains a pressing concern due to limited access to skilled birth attendants, inadequate prenatal care, and cultural barriers that hinder maternal healthcare utilization.

Under-five Mortality Rate: The under-five mortality rate (U5MR) captures the deaths per 1,000 live births among children under five. High U5MR indicates challenges in child health, including malnutrition, preventable diseases, and inadequate healthcare access.

Infant Mortality Rate: The infant mortality rate (IMR) measures the deaths per 1,000 live births among infants under one year of age. High IMR reflects the vulnerability of infants to diseases and health disparities, highlighting the importance of early interventions and maternal health support.

Child Malnutrition: The child malnutrition rates, including stunted growth, wasting, and underweight, provide critical insights into nutrition and food security challenges communities face. Malnutrition compromises children's growth and development, leading to long-term health consequences.

Access to Safe Water and Sanitation: The availability of safe drinking water and sanitation facilities is essential for preventing waterborne diseases and promoting community health. In developing nations, inadequate access to clean water and sanitation remains a significant public health challenge.

Prevalent Diseases

The prevalence of diseases weaves a narrative that transcends borders, cultures, and socio-economic divides. The burden of disease is a stark reminder of the challenges humanity faces in its pursuit of well-being and prosperity, especially in the dynamic landscape of developing nations. It is important to note that the prevalence of these diseases can vary widely by region and country. Public health efforts in developing nations often focus on prevention, early detection, and improving healthcare infrastructure to address these health challenges. Here is a list of some prevalent diseases that are often significant health concerns in developing nations:

Communicable Diseases (CDs): Developing nations often bear a disproportionate burden of infectious diseases that contribute to high morbidity and mortality rates. Malaria, tuberculosis, HIV/AIDS, and neglected tropical diseases are among the prevalent infectious diseases in these regions. In children, CDs like diarrhoea, pneumonia, and vaccine-preventable illnesses significantly contribute to child morbidity and mortality in developing nations. Thus, addressing these CDs requires comprehensive immunization programs, nutrition interventions, and improved healthcare access for children. Factors such as limited healthcare resources, lack of disease surveillance, and challenges in treatment access exacerbate the impact of these diseases.

Non-Communicable Diseases (NCDs): As lifestyles change and populations age, NCDs become increasingly prevalent in developing nations. Cardiovascular diseases, diabetes, cancer, and chronic respiratory illnesses significantly contribute to the NCD burden. Lifestyle factors, including poor nutrition, physical inactivity, and tobacco use, drive the rise of NCDs in these regions.

Neglected Tropical Diseases (NTDs): NTDs affect millions in developing nations, particularly those in poverty-stricken areas. These diseases, including leishmaniasis, schistosomiasis, and lymphatic filariasis, often go unnoticed and untreated, perpetuating the cycle of poverty and ill health.

In understanding these key health indicators and prevalent diseases, policymakers and public health professionals can prioritize interventions, allocate resources strategically, and design targeted programs to address the pressing health challenges in developing nations. Pursuing health equity demands a comprehensive approach that considers the unique contexts, social determinants, and cultural nuances that influence health outcomes in these regions. Through evidence-based strategies and collaborative efforts, we can work towards a healthier future where all communities thrive, irrespective of economic circumstances.

Socioeconomic Factors Influencing Public Health

Public health in developing nations is intricately intertwined with a web of socioeconomic factors that shape the health status and well-being of populations. These factors play a pivotal role in determining access to healthcare, nutrition, education, and overall living conditions. In this section, we explore the critical socioeconomic determinants influencing public health outcomes in developing nations and highlight the importance of addressing these disparities to achieve health equity [3, 4]. Table **2.2** shows examples of socioeconomic factors that influence public health.

Table 2.2. Socioeconomic (SE) factors influencing public health.

S. No.	SE Factors	Remark
1.	Income and Economic Status	Higher-income individuals tend to have better access to healthcare, nutrition, and living conditions. Lower income can lead to reduced access to healthcare services and an increased risk of chronic diseases.
2.	Education	Education plays a significant role in health outcomes. Higher levels of education are associated with healthier behaviors, a better understanding of health information, and improved access to job opportunities with health benefits.
3.	Employment and Job Security	Employment status can affect access to healthcare, as individuals with stable jobs are more likely to have health insurance. Job insecurity and unemployment can lead to increased stress and poor mental health.
4.	Access to Healthcare	Socioeconomic factors can determine access to healthcare services, including insurance coverage, availability of healthcare providers, and affordability of healthcare treatments.
5.	Housing and Neighborhood Conditions	Poor housing conditions, such as overcrowding and inadequate sanitation, can lead to the spread of diseases. Living in neighborhoods with limited access to fresh food, safe parks, and healthcare facilities can also impact health.
6.	Social Support and Networks	Strong social networks and support systems can contribute to better mental and physical health. Conversely, social isolation and lack of social support can lead to poorer health outcomes.
7.	Nutrition and Food Security	Socioeconomic status affects access to nutritious food. Food insecurity, which is more common among lower-income populations, can lead to malnutrition and various health problems.
8.	Environmental Exposures	Socioeconomic factors may influence exposure to environmental hazards, such as pollution and toxins, which are associated with adverse health effects.
9.	Health Behaviors	Socioeconomic status can influence health-related behaviors such as smoking, alcohol consumption, physical activity, and diet. Lower-income individuals may be more likely to engage in unhealthy behaviors due to stress and limited resources.
10.	Access to Education and Health Literacy	Limited access to education and lower health literacy can lead to difficulties in understanding and following healthcare recommendations, resulting in poorer health outcomes.

(Table 2.2) cont.....

S. No.	SE Factors	Remark
11.	Access to Transportation	Lack of transportation options can hinder access to healthcare services, employment, and other essential resources, impacting overall health and well-being.
12.	Racial and Ethnic Disparities	Socioeconomic factors intersect with racial and ethnic disparities in health. Minority populations often face higher rates of poverty, discrimination, and reduced access to healthcare services.

Poverty and Inequality

Poverty is a defining characteristic of many developing nations and casts a long shadow over public health. Impoverished communities face numerous challenges, including limited access to healthcare, inadequate nutrition, and precarious living conditions. Poverty creates barriers to essential health services, preventive care, and disease management, leading to higher morbidity and mortality rates. Additionally, income inequality further exacerbates health disparities, with marginalized populations experiencing worse health outcomes than more privileged groups.

Access to Healthcare

Limited access to healthcare is a persistent challenge in many developing nations, particularly in rural and remote areas. Inadequate healthcare infrastructure, shortage of healthcare professionals, and barriers to healthcare utilization hinder timely access to medical services. Affordability of healthcare also remains a significant concern, as out-of-pocket expenses can be burdensome for families with limited financial resources. Addressing healthcare access gaps requires strengthening health systems, investing in healthcare facilities, and promoting community-based healthcare solutions.

Education and Health Literacy

Education plays a crucial role in shaping health outcomes. A lack of education can limit individuals' understanding of health practices, disease prevention, and healthcare resources. Health literacy, or the ability to access, understand, and apply health information, is vital for making informed decisions about one's health. Low health literacy levels can impede disease prevention efforts, hinder timely healthcare-seeking behaviour, and exacerbate health disparities.

Nutrition and Food Security

Nutrition is a cornerstone of public health, and food insecurity is prevalent in many developing nations. Insufficient access to nutritious food contributes to malnutrition, stunting, and other health problems, especially among children and vulnerable populations. Food security challenges are often exacerbated by environmental factors, climate change, and economic instability. Addressing food insecurity requires a multifaceted approach, including promoting sustainable agriculture, improving food distribution systems, and implementing nutrition education programs.

Sanitation and Access to Clean Water

Inadequate sanitation facilities and lack of access to clean water sources contribute to various health issues in developing nations. Poor sanitation can spread waterborne diseases, such as diarrhoea and cholera, while contaminated water poses significant health risks. Promoting sanitation practices, improving water infrastructure, and implementing water purification initiatives are essential to ensure community health and well-being.

Environmental Factors

Environmental conditions, such as air pollution, exposure to toxins, and natural disasters, significantly impact public health in developing nations. Air pollution, often linked to industrialisation and urbanisation, contributes to respiratory diseases and other health complications. Exposure to environmental toxins, such as heavy metals and pesticides, can also have long-term health effects. Moreover, natural disasters like floods and earthquakes can cause widespread devastation and disrupt healthcare services, exacerbating health vulnerabilities.

Understanding and addressing the socioeconomic factors that influence public health in developing nations are critical steps towards achieving health equity and improving overall well-being. Sustainable progress requires collaborative efforts from governments, non-governmental organisations, international agencies, and local communities to address disparities, strengthen healthcare systems, and promote policies prioritising all individuals' health and dignity. By investing in holistic approaches that tackle these determinants, we can pave the way for healthier, more resilient communities and foster a brighter future for generations to come.

Health Disparities, Inequities and Equity

In the diverse tapestry of developing nations, health disparities and inequities form a stark reality affecting populations' well-being across socioeconomic strata. These disparities, driven by various factors, create unequal access to healthcare, nutrition, education, and other essential determinants of health. This section delves into the complex nature of health disparities, inequities, and equity, exploring their root causes, consequences, and the imperative of addressing them to create just and inclusive health systems [5, 6].

Root Causes of Health Disparities

Health disparities in developing nations are multifactorial, rooted in a combination of social, economic, and cultural determinants. Poverty, limited access to healthcare services, inadequate education, and food insecurity are among the key contributors to health disparities. Additionally, gender inequalities, discrimination based on ethnicity or caste, and geographic isolation can further exacerbate disparities, leading to differential health outcomes for marginalized populations.

Access to Healthcare

Unequal access to healthcare services remains a fundamental driver of health disparities in developing nations. Rural and remote areas often face challenges in healthcare infrastructure and a shortage of healthcare professionals, leading to limited access to medical care. Financial barriers, including out-of-pocket expenses for healthcare, can deter individuals from seeking necessary treatment, exacerbating health disparities between the affluent and vulnerable populations.

Maternal and Child Health

Health disparities in maternal and child health are particularly concerning in developing nations. Women and children from disadvantaged backgrounds often face greater risks during pregnancy and childbirth due to limited access to skilled birth attendants, prenatal care, and maternal health support. The lack of essential healthcare interventions, such as immunization and nutrition programs, can result in higher infant mortality rates and childhood illnesses among vulnerable communities.

Infectious Diseases

Infectious diseases disproportionately affect underserved communities, contributing to health disparities in developing nations. Factors such as overcrowded living conditions, inadequate sanitation, and limited access to healthcare facilities can increase the risk of disease transmission. Communities with reduced access to preventive measures, such as vaccinations and disease surveillance, are more vulnerable to outbreaks of infectious diseases, leading to higher morbidity and mortality rates.

Non-Communicable Diseases (NCDs)

The burden of non-communicable diseases (NCDs) also contributes to health disparities in developing nations. Lifestyle-related risk factors, such as poor nutrition, physical inactivity, and tobacco use, are more prevalent among disadvantaged populations, driving the rise of NCDs in these regions. Limited access to healthcare for early detection and management of NCDs further widens health inequities.

Mental Health

Mental health disparities are often overlooked in developing nations, where stigma and limited resources create significant barriers to mental health services. Vulnerable populations, including women, children, and refugees, are at heightened risk of mental health challenges due to adverse living conditions, trauma, and social isolation. Addressing mental health disparities requires integrating mental health services into primary care, raising awareness, and reducing the stigma surrounding mental illness.

Consequences of Health Disparities

Health disparities have far-reaching consequences on both individuals and communities. They perpetuate a cycle of poverty and ill health, hindering socio-economic development and human potential. Disadvantaged individuals often face reduced life expectancy, increased morbidity, and decreased quality of life. Moreover, health disparities significantly burden healthcare systems, impeding progress in achieving universal health coverage and sustainable development goals.

The Imperative of Health Equity

Achieving health equity in developing nations is an urgent moral, public health, and social justice imperative. Health equity recognizes that each individual deserves the right to attain the highest possible standard of health, regardless of their social, economic, or geographic circumstances. In contrast to equality, which assumes that everyone starts from the same place and needs the same resources, equity accounts for the uneven playing field and works to level it by addressing the underlying causes of disparities.

To promote health equity, it is crucial to implement multi-faceted interventions that prioritize vulnerable populations, strengthen healthcare systems, and foster inclusive policies that account for the social determinants of health.

The journey towards equity requires collaboration among governments, non-governmental organizations, communities, and international agencies. Together, these efforts can reduce the structural barriers that perpetuate inequities, ensuring that every individual has access to quality healthcare and an equal chance to live a healthy, fulfilling life.

Case Study 1: *Improving Maternal and Child Health in Rural Country X.*

In rural country X, high maternal and child mortality rates posed significant public health challenges. Limited access to skilled birth attendants and maternal health services led to avoidable complications during childbirth, resulting in maternal deaths and increased neonatal mortality. To address these disparities, a community-based initiative was launched involving local healthcare workers, community leaders, and non-governmental organizations.

The initiative focused on enhancing maternal health awareness, promoting antenatal care, and facilitating safe deliveries. Community health workers were trained to provide prenatal support, conduct health education sessions, and identify high-risk pregnancies for referral. Additionally, mobile health clinics were set up to deliver essential care to remote communities. Through community engagement and empowerment, women were encouraged to participate actively in their maternal health journey, making informed decisions about childbirth and adopting healthy practices.

Over time, the initiative yielded promising results. Maternal mortality rates significantly decreased, and the percentage of women accessing antenatal care increased. Neonatal mortality also declined, reflecting improved maternal health and access to essential newborn care. The success of this initiative highlighted the transformative potential of community-driven interventions in addressing maternal and child health disparities in resource-limited settings.

Case Study 2: *Combating HIV/AIDS in Sub-Saharan Africa through Community-Based Programs.*

Sub-Saharan Africa has been heavily affected by the HIV/AIDS pandemic, with millions of people living with the virus. In many communities, stigma and misconceptions surrounding HIV/AIDS hindered prevention efforts and access to treatment. To combat the epidemic, community-based programs were established to address the root causes of health disparities and engage affected populations.

Local non-governmental organizations partnered with healthcare providers, community leaders, and people living with HIV/AIDS to design comprehensive prevention, testing, and treatment initiatives. These programs focused on raising awareness, reducing stigma, and ensuring equitable access to antiretroviral therapy. Community health workers played a crucial role in reaching remote areas, providing counseling, and offering support to affected individuals and families.

The impact of these community-based programs was significant. HIV testing rates increased, leading to earlier diagnosis and treatment initiation. The proportion of people living with HIV who were virally suppressed rose, contributing to reduced transmission rates. Moreover, by integrating HIV/AIDS care with other health services, the programs helped to address the broader health needs of affected communities.

These case studies exemplify the power of community engagement and empowerment in addressing public health challenges in developing nations. By leveraging local knowledge, resources, and resilience, community-based initiatives can drive transformative change, leading to healthier and more equitable societies.

CONCLUSION

In tackling health disparities, inequities, and the broader goal of health equity, it becomes clear that addressing the diverse and complex challenges of public health in developing nations requires a holistic and inclusive approach. By thoroughly understanding key health indicators, prevalent diseases, and socioeconomic determinants, we can create interventions that not only address immediate health disparities but also promote long-term equity. Through collaborative efforts and dedicated partnerships, we can work toward a future where health equity is a reality, ensuring that no one is left behind due to their socioeconomic circumstances.

REFERENCES

[1]   World Health Organization. World Health Statistics 2021: Monitoring Health for the SDGs. World Health Organization, 2021. Available from: https://www.who.int/publications/i/item/9789240027053

[2]   Institute for Health Metrics and Evaluation (IHME). Global Burden of Disease Study 2019 (GBD 2019) Results. IHME, University of Washington, 2021. Available from: https://vizhub.healthdata.org/gbd-results/

[3]   Marmot, M. The Health Gap: The Challenge of an Unequal World. Bloomsbury Publishing, 2020. ISBN: 978-1632863788.

[4]   Braveman P, Gottlieb L. The social determinants of health: it's time to consider the causes of the causes. Public Health Rep 2014; 129(1_suppl2): 19-31.
        [http://dx.doi.org/10.1177/00333549141291S206] [PMID: 24385661]

[5]   World Health Organization. A conceptual framework for action on the social determinants of health. Social Determinants of Health Discussion Paper 2 (Policy and Practice), 2010. Available from: https://apps.who.int/iris/handle/10665/44489

[6]   World Health Organization. Regional Office for Europe. The WHO European health equity status report initiative: understanding the drivers of health equity: the power of political participation. World Health Organization. Regional Office for Europe, 2020. Available from: https://apps.who.int/iris/handle/10665/337952

CHAPTER 3

Building Resilience in Developing Communities

Abstract: Resilience in public health is crucial for communities facing diverse health challenges in developing nations. This chapter explores the concept of resilience, factors contributing to community resilience, and case studies showcasing successful resilience-building initiatives. By understanding and fostering resilience, communities can effectively withstand and recover from health adversities, ultimately promoting well-being and sustainability.

Keywords: Adaptability, Collaboration, Community engagement, Developing communities, Early warning systems, Healthcare infrastructure, Public health, Resilience.

INTRODUCTION

Resilience in public health refers to communities' capacity to withstand, adapt, and thrive amidst health challenges. It encompasses proactive measures, community strengths, and response mechanisms to navigate adversities effectively. Key elements include robust health infrastructure, community engagement, prevention, preparedness, and addressing health disparities.

Building resilience in developing communities requires a multifaceted approach. Strong social networks, community engagement, accessible healthcare infrastructure, early warning systems, education, collaboration, flexibility, empathy, and cultural preservation are essential factors contributing to resilience. These elements empower communities to respond effectively to health crises and promote well-being.

Defining Resilience in the Context of Public Health

Resilience, in the context of public health, is a dynamic and multifaceted concept that embodies the capacity of communities and individuals to withstand, adapt, and thrive in the face of adversity, particularly in the realm of health challenges. It is an approach that acknowledges the inevitability of setbacks and disruptions, recognizing that building preparedness and response mechanisms is essential in navigating the uncertainties of the future [1, 2].

In the public health context, resilience extends beyond mere survival; it encompasses the ability to rebound and grow stronger in the aftermath of health crises. Resilient communities draw upon their inherent strengths, social networks, and adaptive capacities to proactively address health disparities, prevent diseases, and promote well-being [1, 2].

Elements of Resilience

Resilience in public health is shaped by a combination of interconnected elements that foster community well-being and response readiness:

Health Infrastructure: A robust and well-functioning health infrastructure is the backbone of resilient communities. Adequate healthcare facilities, skilled healthcare professionals, and efficient healthcare systems are essential in responding to health emergencies effectively.

Community Engagement: Engaging communities actively in shaping public health initiatives is crucial for resilience. When community members have a sense of ownership and empowerment, they are more invested in designing and implementing sustainable health interventions.

Prevention and Preparedness: Resilient communities prioritize prevention and preparedness strategies, anticipating and mitigating health risks before they escalate into crises. Early detection, surveillance systems, and health education are vital in building resilience.

Social Cohesion: Strong social bonds and support networks within communities enhance resilience. Social cohesion fosters mutual aid, collective problem-solving, and emotional support during health crises.

Adaptability and Flexibility: Resilient communities display adaptability and flexibility in responding to health challenges. They can adjust strategies and resources to suit changing circumstances and evolving health threats.

Knowledge and Education: Access to accurate health information and education empowers communities to make informed decisions about their health. Knowledge equips individuals with the tools to prevent diseases, seek appropriate care, and adopt healthy practices.

Navigating Health Disparities

Resilience in public health becomes particularly critical in navigating health disparities that are prevalent in developing nations. Disadvantaged communities often face multiple health challenges due to social, economic, and environmental factors. Resilient approaches acknowledge these disparities and seek to address the root causes to achieve health equity.

Resilient communities focus on bridging gaps in healthcare access and reducing barriers to preventive measures, ensuring that vulnerable populations receive equitable health services. By prioritizing the needs of marginalized groups and integrating their perspectives into public health initiatives, resilience aims to level the playing field and create a more equitable healthcare landscape.

The Role of Preparedness in Resilience

Preparedness is a cornerstone of resilience in public health. Being prepared involves anticipating and planning for potential health threats, such as disease outbreaks, natural disasters, and environmental hazards. Robust preparedness measures involve developing response protocols, stockpiling essential resources, and training healthcare professionals and community members in emergency response.

When communities are prepared, they can mobilize swiftly and efficiently during crises, minimizing the impact on health and well-being. Preparedness efforts also extend to establishing communication networks, ensuring the dissemination of accurate information during emergencies, and fostering collaboration between various stakeholders.

In summary, resilience in the context of public health is a proactive and adaptive approach that empowers communities to confront health challenges with strength and determination. It encompasses a wide array of elements, from healthcare infrastructure and community engagement to prevention, preparedness, and social cohesion. Resilient communities recognize the importance of addressing health disparities and promoting health equity, aiming to create a more inclusive and sustainable healthcare landscape for all. By embracing resilience, developing communities can forge a path towards a healthier and more equitable future.

Factors Contributing to Community Resilience

Building resilience in developing communities is a multifaceted endeavour that draws strength from various factors working in harmony. These contributing elements are pivotal in enhancing community preparedness, response capabilities, and adaptive capacities to navigate public health challenges. In this section, we explore the key factors that contribute to community resilience and foster the ability of communities to withstand and recover from health adversities [3 - 5].

Strong Social Networks and Community Cohesion

At the core of community resilience lies the strength of social networks and community cohesion. Strong social bonds facilitate mutual support, resource-sharing, and collective problem-solving during times of crisis. Social networks act as information channels, ensuring vital health information reaches all community members promptly. A tightly knit community is more likely to collaborate and mobilize resources effectively, fostering resilience in the face of health challenges.

Community Engagement and Empowerment

Community engagement and empowerment are critical factors in building resilience. When communities are actively involved in the decision-making process regarding public health interventions, they develop a sense of ownership and accountability. Empowered communities are more likely to take proactive steps to address health disparities, promote preventive practices, and advocate for their health needs. Engaged communities collaborate with public health agencies, local governments, and non-governmental organizations, co-creating resilient solutions that align with their unique needs and context.

Accessible and Responsive Healthcare Infrastructure

Resilient communities rely on a healthcare infrastructure that is accessible, well-functioning, and responsive to their health needs. Adequate healthcare facilities, equipped with essential resources and skilled healthcare professionals, form the backbone of resilience. Access to quality healthcare services, including preventive care, early detection, and treatment, strengthens a community's capacity to manage health challenges effectively.

Early Warning Systems and Surveillance

Timely detection of health threats is paramount for building resilience. Early warning systems and surveillance mechanisms enable communities to promptly identify and respond to potential health crises. Monitoring disease trends, outbreaks, and environmental risks empowers communities to take proactive measures and allocate resources to prevent escalation.

Education and Health Literacy

Education plays a transformative role in fostering resilience. Health literacy equips individuals with the knowledge and skills needed to make informed decisions about their health. Education about disease prevention, healthy practices, and proper healthcare utilization empowers communities to adopt proactive measures and promote well-being.

Collaboration and Partnerships

Resilience is not a solitary pursuit; it thrives on collaboration and partnerships between diverse stakeholders. Governments, non-governmental organizations, international agencies, and local community-based organizations play complementary roles in fostering resilience. These partnerships can create comprehensive and sustainable health interventions by combining resources, expertise, and capacities.

Flexibility and Adaptability

Resilient communities exhibit flexibility and adaptability in the face of ever-changing health challenges. They can adjust strategies, reallocate resources, and leverage innovative approaches to respond effectively to crises. Adaptability allows communities to learn from past experiences and continuously improve their preparedness for future adversities.

Empathy and Psychological Support

Psychological support is essential in building resilience, especially during times of crisis. Empathy and emotional support strengthen individuals and communities, enabling them to cope with stress, trauma, and loss. Initiatives that prioritize mental health, counselling services, and trauma-informed care foster community well-being and enhance resilience.

Cultural Preservation and Traditional Knowledge

Preserving cultural heritage and traditional knowledge is instrumental in building resilience. Indigenous practices and traditional healing methods often hold valuable insights into preventive healthcare and community well-being. Integrating cultural values and practices into public health interventions fosters trust and community engagement.

In conclusion, community resilience in developing nations draws its strength from diverse factors encompassing social cohesion, community empowerment, accessible healthcare infrastructure, early warning systems, education, and collaboration. Embracing flexibility, adaptability, empathy, and cultural preservation enhances a community's capacity to navigate public health challenges and emerge stronger in adversity. By fostering these contributing elements, stakeholders can work together to empower communities, promote health equity, and build a future where resilience is a cornerstone of public health.

In conclusion, these case studies exemplify the power of community resilience in the face of health challenges. In both instances, community engagement, empowerment, early detection, and collaboration with external stakeholders played crucial roles in overcoming health adversities. Resilient communities demonstrate that leveraging their inherent strengths, engaging in proactive health initiatives, and fostering partnerships can build a healthier and more sustainable future for all. The lessons learned from these case studies can inspire other developing communities seeking to build resilience in their public health landscapes.

Case Study 3: *Resilient Response to Cholera Outbreak in a Rural Village in Country X*

In a remote rural village in Country X, access to healthcare and sanitation facilities was limited, making the community vulnerable to disease outbreaks. In 2022, a cholera outbreak struck the region, posing a severe public health challenge. Despite facing adversities, the community responded with resilience and unity, demonstrating the power of collective action in crisis management. The key factors that contributed to resilience are:

• *Community Engagement and Empowerment:* Community leaders and local health workers actively engaged with the villagers, disseminating critical information about cholera prevention and early signs of infection. The community members were empowered to take ownership of their health by participating in hygiene education programs and implementing safe water and sanitation practices.
• *Early Detection and Response:* Recognizing the importance of early detection, the village established a simple but effective surveillance system. Local health workers were trained to identify and report cholera cases promptly. This early warning system allowed for swift response measures to contain the outbreak.
• *Strengthening Healthcare Infrastructure:* The community collaborated with a local healthcare organization to establish a temporary clinic to isolate and treat cholera patients. The clinic was equipped with basic medical supplies, and health professionals from neighboring regions volunteered to support the efforts.
• *Social Cohesion and Mutual Support:* The community displayed remarkable social cohesion, supporting the affected families and those working in the temporary clinic. Neighbors shared resources, provided emotional support, and volunteered to care for children and elders, allowing healthcare workers to focus on treating patients.

Outcome: Through the collaborative efforts of the government and community champions and external support led by the World Health Organization, the cholera outbreak was contained within a few months. The number of cases decreased significantly, and no new infections were reported after the initial response phase. The village's resilience in the face of the outbreak showcased the potential of community-driven initiatives and the importance of empowering communities to take charge of their health.

Case Study 4: *Building Resilience against Malaria in a Rural Community in Country X*

In a rural community in country X, malaria was a persistent health threat, causing significant morbidity and mortality, particularly among children and pregnant women. The community recognized the urgency of addressing this burden and embraced a resilient approach to combat malaria. The key factors that contributed to resilience are:

- *Prevention and Health Education:* The community launched an extensive health education campaign, raising awareness about malaria transmission, prevention methods, and the importance of seeking timely treatment. Informational sessions were held regularly, and community health workers were trained to distribute mosquito nets and educate families on their proper use.
- *Engaging Youth and Women:* The community actively engaged youth and women in the fight against malaria. Youth-led initiatives organized cleanup campaigns to eliminate mosquito breeding sites, while women's groups distributed mosquito nets and organized health check-ups for pregnant women to monitor their health and ensure early detection and treatment of malaria.
- *Strengthening Healthcare Facilities:* Recognizing the need for accessible healthcare, the community collaborated with a local health organization and government agencies to strengthen healthcare facilities. The healthcare center received essential medical supplies, malaria testing kits, and anti-malarial medications to improve the quality of care.
- *Traditional Medicine Integration:* The community acknowledged the significance of traditional medicine in managing malaria symptoms. Traditional healers were engaged in the education campaign and were encouraged to work collaboratively with modern healthcare providers to ensure appropriate treatment and care.

Outcome: Over time, the community's resilience against malaria resulted in a significant reduction in malaria cases. The implementation of preventive measures, such as the proper use of mosquito nets and environmental cleanup, led to a decline in mosquito breeding sites. Timely access to healthcare and early detection of malaria cases further contributed to improved health outcomes. The community's strong social ties and collaboration with government and agencies fostered sustainable strategies to combat malaria.

CONCLUSION

Building resilience in developing communities is essential for addressing health challenges and promoting sustainable development. By embracing community engagement, strengthening healthcare infrastructure, fostering collaboration, and prioritizing preparedness, communities can effectively navigate health adversities and emerge stronger. The case studies exemplify successful resilience-building initiatives, emphasizing the importance of proactive measures and community empowerment. Through collective efforts, stakeholders can foster a future where resilience is ingrained in public health systems, ensuring the well-being of all individuals and communities.

REFERENCES

[1]   Norris FH, Stevens SP, Pfefferbaum B, Wyche KF, Pfefferbaum RL. Community resilience as a metaphor, theory, set of capacities, and strategy for disaster readiness. Am J Community Psychol 2008; 41(1-2): 127-50.
[http://dx.doi.org/10.1007/s10464-007-9156-6] [PMID: 18157631]

[2]   Luthar SS, Cicchetti D, Becker B. The construct of resilience: a critical evaluation and guidelines for future work. Child Dev 2000; 71(3): 543-62.
[http://dx.doi.org/10.1111/1467-8624.00164] [PMID: 10953923]

[3]   Aldrich DP, Meyer MA. Social capital and community resilience. Am Behav Sci 2015; 59(2): 254-69.
[http://dx.doi.org/10.1177/0002764214550299]

[4]   Cunsolo A, Ellis NR. Ecological grief as a mental health response to climate change-related loss. Nat Clim Chang 2018; 8(4): 275-81.
[http://dx.doi.org/10.1038/s41558-018-0092-2]

[5]   Ungar M. Social ecologies and their contribution to resilience. In: Ungar M, Ed. The Social Ecology of Resilience. New York: Springer 2012; pp. 13-31.
[http://dx.doi.org/10.1007/978-1-4614-0586-3_2]

CHAPTER 4

Inclusive and Equitable Public Health Partnerships

Abstract: Community engagement in public health decision-making is essential for effective and sustainable interventions in developing nations. This chapter explores the principles and practices of community-based participatory approaches, focusing on engaging communities, promoting inclusivity and equity, and strengthening partnerships with stakeholders. By involving communities as active partners, addressing health disparities, and fostering collaborative relationships, public health interventions can achieve greater impact and resilience.

Keywords: Community-based participatory approach, Community engagement, Equity, Inclusivity, Partnerships, Stakeholders.

INTRODUCTION

Engaging communities in public health decision-making is crucial for the success and sustainability of interventions. This section discusses the benefits, key components, and challenges of community engagement, emphasizing the importance of inclusive representation, collaborative planning, capacity building, effective communication, and overcoming barriers to participation.

Promoting inclusivity and equity in public health interventions is essential for addressing health disparities and building resilient communities. This section highlights strategies for recognizing and addressing health disparities, ensuring culturally competent interventions, language accessibility, tailored outreach, empowering marginalized groups, data collection, and engaging local partners.

Effective community partnerships with stakeholders are pivotal for successful public health interventions. This section explores the identification of key stakeholders, fostering collaborative decision-making, sharing resources and expertise, building capacity and training, advocating for sustainable support, monitoring and evaluation, recognition, acknowledgment, building trust, and maintaining long-term relationships.

Engaging Communities in Public Health Decision-Making

In pursuing effective and sustainable public health interventions, community engagement is a pivotal aspect that underpins the success of initiatives in developing nations. Engaging communities in public health decision-making is a transformative approach recognizing community members' expertise, knowledge, and unique perspectives. By involving them as active partners in the design, implementation, and evaluation of public health programs, this participatory approach fosters ownership, empowerment, and community-driven solutions that address the population's health needs more effectively [1, 2].

The Benefits of Community Engagement in Public Health

Engaging communities in public health decision-making yields a myriad of benefits that contribute to the success and sustainability of interventions:

- *Culturally Relevant Interventions:* Communities have intricate knowledge of cultural norms, values, and practices. By involving them in decision-making, public health interventions become more culturally sensitive and contextually relevant, increasing the likelihood of community acceptance and adoption.
- *Tailored Interventions:* Community members deeply understand their health challenges and needs. Their participation allows public health professionals to tailor interventions that directly address the specific issues faced by the community, ensuring resources are directed where they are most needed.
- *Enhanced Health Outcomes:* Engaging communities empowers individuals to take charge of their health. By actively participating in decision-making, they become more invested in the success of the interventions, leading to better adherence to preventive practices, treatment regimens, and healthier lifestyle choices.
- *Improved Utilization of Services:* When communities are involved in decision-making, they gain trust in the healthcare system. This trust can increase healthcare-seeking behavior, as community members are more likely to access and utilize health services when they feel heard and respected.
- *Strengthened Community Cohesion:* Community engagement fosters a sense of unity and shared responsibility for health outcomes. Collaborative decision-making processes strengthen social cohesion and create an environment of mutual support and collective action during health crises.
- *Sustainable Solutions:* Community-driven interventions are more likely to be sustainable in the long term. When community members actively participate in decision-making, they become invested in the success of the programs and are more motivated to maintain and adapt the initiatives as needed.

Key Components of Community Engagement

Effective community engagement in public health decision-making requires a thoughtful and inclusive approach. Key components of community engagement include:

- *Inclusive Representation:* Ensure diverse representation from different subgroups within the community, including marginalized populations, women, youth, and elders. This representation fosters inclusivity and allows for a comprehensive understanding of community needs.
- *Collaborative Planning:* Collaborate with community members from the outset of the planning process. Engage in open discussions, share information, and jointly identify health priorities and goals.
- *Capacity Building:* Provide training and capacity-building opportunities to community members to enhance their understanding of public health concepts, data analysis, and advocacy skills. Empowered individuals are better equipped to participate effectively in decision-making.
- *Effective Communication:* Foster clear and transparent communication channels to ensure that information flows freely between public health professionals and community members. Utilize culturally appropriate communication methods to disseminate information effectively.
- *Respect for Local Knowledge:* Respect and value the local knowledge, practices, and traditional healing methods that community members bring to the table. Collaborate with traditional healers and community leaders to integrate traditional practices with modern healthcare.

Overcoming Challenges in Community Engagement

While community engagement is invaluable, it may face certain challenges that need to be addressed:

- *Time and Resource Constraints:* Engaging communities in decision-making requires time and resources. Public health professionals and organizations need to allocate sufficient resources and be prepared for the time investment required for effective community engagement.
- *Language and Cultural Barriers:* Overcoming language and cultural barriers is essential for meaningful engagement. Translators and cultural brokers can facilitate effective communication and understanding.
- *Power Dynamics:* Power imbalances can hinder meaningful engagement. Public health professionals must recognize and address these dynamics to ensure equitable participation from all community members.

- *Sustainability:* Maintaining community engagement over the long term can be challenging. Efforts should be made to institutionalize community engagement practices within public health systems to ensure sustainability.

In conclusion, community engagement in public health decision-making is a powerful tool that fosters collaborative, contextually relevant, and sustainable interventions in developing nations. By embracing a participatory approach, public health professionals can harness the knowledge, strengths, and aspirations of communities, co-creating a path towards improved health outcomes and equitable well-being for all.

Promoting Inclusivity and Equity in Interventions

In the pursuit of building resilient communities and addressing public health challenges in developing nations, promoting inclusivity and equity in interventions is essential. An inclusive approach ensures that the diverse needs, perspectives, and voices of all community members are recognized and valued in decision-making processes. Equity, on the other hand, addresses the disparities and injustices that exist within communities, seeking to provide fair opportunities and resources to improve health outcomes for everyone. Public health interventions can foster social justice, reduce health disparities, and strengthen community resilience by promoting inclusivity and equity [3, 4].

Recognizing and Addressing Health Disparities

To promote inclusivity and equity, it is crucial to identify and address health disparities within the community. Vulnerable populations, such as women, children, the elderly, people with disabilities, and marginalized ethnic or socioeconomic groups, may face unique challenges that require tailored interventions. Understanding the root causes of disparities, such as poverty, discrimination, and limited access to resources, is essential in designing targeted strategies to bridge the gaps in health outcomes.

Culturally Competent Interventions

Inclusive interventions must be culturally competent, considering the cultural norms, beliefs, and practices of the community. By collaborating with community members and cultural brokers, public health professionals can ensure that interventions are sensitive to cultural preferences, language, and social norms. This approach enhances community acceptance and engagement, leading to greater effectiveness and sustainability of the interventions.

Language Accessibility and Communication

Language can be a significant barrier to inclusivity in public health interventions. Providing information in the community's primary language is crucial to ensure that all members understand the interventions, their benefits, and how to access them. Utilizing clear and accessible communication methods, such as visual aids and community meetings, fosters effective communication and active participation.

Tailored Outreach and Accessibility

To promote equity, interventions should be designed to reach the most vulnerable and underserved populations. Tailored outreach efforts can include bringing healthcare services directly to remote areas, offering transportation support, and conducting health campaigns in places accessible to all community members. Removing financial barriers and ensuring that interventions are affordable and accessible to all are essential for equitable health outcomes.

Empowering Marginalized Groups

Empowering marginalized groups is a key strategy to promote inclusivity and equity. Initiatives that actively involve women, youth, people with disabilities, and other marginalized communities in decision-making and leadership roles enhance their sense of agency and promote their health and well-being. By involving these groups in planning and implementing interventions, their unique needs and concerns are prioritized.

Data Collection and Evaluation

Collecting disaggregated data helps identify disparities and inequities within the community. Data that captures the experiences and health outcomes of different population groups allows public health professionals to monitor progress, evaluate the effectiveness of interventions, and make evidence-based decisions to promote inclusivity and equity.

Engaging Local Partners and Stakeholders

Engaging local partners and stakeholders is instrumental in promoting inclusivity and equity. Collaborating with community-based organizations, local leaders, and non-governmental organizations ensures that interventions are contextually relevant and align with community priorities. Local partnerships also build trust and foster sustainable relationships with the community.

In conclusion, promoting inclusivity and equity in public health interventions is central to building resilient communities and addressing health challenges in developing nations. By acknowledging and addressing health disparities, providing culturally competent and accessible interventions, empowering marginalized groups, and engaging with local partners, public health professionals can foster social justice, reduce health inequalities, and strengthen the fabric of community-based participatory approaches. Embracing inclusivity and equity ensures that no one is left behind and that public health interventions lead to a more equitable and healthier future for all community members.

Strengthening Community Partnerships with Stakeholders

Effective community partnerships with stakeholders are pivotal in building resilient communities and driving successful public health interventions in developing nations. These partnerships foster collaboration, resource-sharing, and collective action, leveraging the expertise and contributions of diverse stakeholders to address complex health challenges. Community-based participatory approaches can thrive by forging solid connections with governments, non-governmental organizations (NGOs), healthcare providers, academia, and the private sector, leading to sustainable and equitable health outcomes [5, 6].

Identifying Key Stakeholders

The first step in strengthening community partnerships is identifying key stakeholders relevant to the specific public health issue. These stakeholders can vary depending on the context and the nature of the intervention. Common stakeholders include:

- *Government Agencies:* Engaging with local, regional, and national government agencies is crucial for policy support, resource allocation, and creating an enabling environment for public health initiatives.
- *Non-Governmental Organizations (NGOs):* NGOs often possess expertise in specific health areas and have established community networks. Partnering with NGOs can enhance intervention reach and effectiveness.
- *Healthcare Providers:* Collaboration with healthcare providers, including hospitals, clinics, and community health workers, enables the integration of healthcare services and expertise into the interventions.
- *Academic Institutions:* Partnering with academic institutions facilitates research collaboration, data analysis, and evidence-based decision-making for interventions.
- *Private Sector:* The private sector can contribute resources, funding, and technical expertise to support public health initiatives.

Fostering Collaborative Decision-Making

Effective community partnerships require collaborative decision-making, where stakeholders work together to design, implement, and evaluate interventions. Engaging stakeholders from the outset is essential for ensuring that interventions are grounded in local realities, respond to the specific needs of the community, and are supported by those most affected. There are two broad ways to consider for effective results:

Engaging Stakeholders from the Beginning

Stakeholder engagement can be achieved through a structured and inclusive process to bring diverse voices to the table, and this involves:

- **Stakeholder Mapping:** Before initiating any project, it is critical to identify the key stakeholders *e.g.*, community leaders, government officials, NGOs, CSOs, healthcare providers, and vulnerable groups. The mapping helps visualize and categorize the stakeholders based on their interests, influence, and potential contribution to the project.
- **Consultative Meetings and Focus Groups:** Organize meetings and focus groups to solicit input from different stakeholders on community needs, priorities, and potential challenges. These consultations can be both formal and informal to encourage broad participation.
- **Needs Assessments:** This involves stakeholders in data collection and analysis of the community's needs. By including stakeholders in this initial phase, the project can accurately reflect the lived experiences of the population.
- **Advisory Committees and Leadership Teams:** Create stakeholder advisory committees that include representatives from various sectors of the community. This committee can help guide decision-making throughout the project lifecycle, ensuring that interventions remain aligned with community needs.

Example 1: In a rural health intervention project, stakeholder mapping might reveal that religious leaders hold significant influence in the community. Involving them as early advocates helps foster trust and support for the project. Alongside this, a series of community forums can be organized to engage women, youth, and marginalized groups, allowing them to share their experiences and ideas for improving maternal health services. To gain a deeper understanding of local challenges, a participatory rural appraisal (PRA) method can be used, where community members actively map out their health service access points, providing insights into barriers and potential solutions. Finally, a multi-stakeholder health advisory board can be established to oversee the implementation of a new vaccination campaign, ensuring continuous feedback from local healthcare workers, community members, and government officials throughout the project lifecycle.

NB: The above example aims to provide a comprehensive view of stakeholder engagement from multiple angles.

Mechanisms to Incentivize Stakeholder Participation

Engaging stakeholders often requires thoughtful incentives to encourage sustained participation. Some mechanisms include:

- **Capacity Building and Skill Development:** Offering training programs or workshops that enhance stakeholders' knowledge and skills can be a strong incentive for involvement. By equipping them with leadership or technical skills, stakeholders become active participants and advocates for the project.
- **Providing Platforms for Influence and Recognition:** Stakeholders are more likely to engage when they feel that their contributions will be recognized and their voices have influence. Providing platforms where they can regularly share their views and contribute to decision-making enhances their commitment.
- **Monetary or In-kind Compensation:** While not always necessary, offering modest stipends, travel reimbursements, or in-kind compensation (*e.g.*, food or tools) can be an effective way to support stakeholder engagement, particularly for those from low-income or vulnerable backgrounds.
- **Social Recognition and Empowerment:** Publicly acknowledging stakeholders' contributions in meetings, reports, or through media channels can build trust and reinforce their importance to the project.
- **Involving Stakeholders in Evaluation:** When stakeholders are involved not just in planning but also in the monitoring and evaluation of interventions, they feel a deeper sense of responsibility and accomplishment.

Example 2: In a rural health project, community health workers can be involved in training programs on disease surveillance, not only strengthening their capacity but also fostering a sense of ownership in the project's success. To keep stakeholders engaged and ensure their voices are heard, regular feedback loops, such as town hall meetings or digital platforms, can be established, allowing participants to provide ongoing input on project progress. Community members who contribute time to facilitate health awareness workshops may be compensated with transportation allowances or small stipends, offering tangible support for their involvement. Additionally, publicly recognizing a community leader's efforts in spearheading a clean water initiative - whether through newsletters or social media - can boost their standing and encourage further participation. Finally, by including community members in data collection and evaluation of health outcomes, they are empowered to directly assess the project's impact and contribute to its long-term improvement.

NB: The above example aims to outline various mechanisms that incentivize participation while building community ownership and involvement.

Sharing Resources and Expertise

Strengthening partnerships involves sharing resources and expertise among stakeholders. Governments can allocate funds and resources, NGOs can provide technical assistance, healthcare providers can deliver services, and academia can contribute research and data analysis. By pooling resources and leveraging each stakeholder's unique strengths, interventions become more comprehensive and sustainable.

Building Capacity and Training

Building the capacity of community members and stakeholders is integral to the success of partnerships. Providing training on public health issues, data collection, community engagement, and leadership skills enhances the effectiveness of interventions and empowers stakeholders to take on meaningful roles.

Advocating for Sustainable Support

Strong community partnerships can advocate for sustainable support from governments and donors. Collaboratively presenting evidence of the intervention's impact and effectiveness can garner ongoing support and resources, ensuring the continuity of public health efforts.

Monitoring and Evaluation

Continuous monitoring and evaluation are essential for the success of community partnerships. Regular assessments help identify strengths and areas for improvement, ensuring that interventions remain responsive to evolving community needs.

Recognition and Acknowledgment

Recognizing and acknowledging the contributions of stakeholders fosters a positive and collaborative working environment. Appreciation for their efforts strengthens the commitment of stakeholders to the success of the intervention.

Building Trust and Long-Term Relationships

Building trust and maintaining long-term relationships are fundamental to sustaining community partnerships. Transparent communication, shared values, and mutual respect are the cornerstones of enduring collaborations.

In conclusion, strengthening community partnerships with stakeholders is pivotal for successful community-based participatory approaches in developing nations. Community partnerships can thrive by identifying key stakeholders, fostering collaborative decision-making, sharing resources and expertise, building capacity, advocating for support, monitoring and evaluating interventions, and building trust, driving sustainable and equitable public health outcomes. Embracing the collective strength of diverse stakeholders, these partnerships pave the way for healthier, resilient communities where health challenges are met with solidarity and innovation.

Case Study 5: *Empowering Women's Health in a Rural Village in Country X*

Context: In a rural village in country X, women faced significant health disparities, including limited access to healthcare services, lack of health education, and high maternal and infant mortality rates. To address these challenges, a community-based participatory approach was adopted, involving community members, local healthcare providers, and a women-led NGO.

Key Components of the Community-Based Participatory Approach:

- Community Engagement: The women of the village took the lead in organizing community meetings and discussions to identify health priorities and challenges. They actively engaged with other community members to ensure diverse perspectives were heard.
- Capacity Building: The women's NGO provided health education and training sessions for the women in the village, focusing on maternal and child health, family planning, and nutrition. This empowered the women with knowledge and skills to make informed decisions about their health.
- Partnership with Healthcare Providers: The local healthcare center collaborated with the women's NGO to conduct regular health check-ups, prenatal care, and immunization drives in the village. This ensured that healthcare services were accessible and tailored to the community's needs.
- Women's Health Committee: A Women's Health Committee was formed, comprising representatives from the village and the NGO. The committee took charge of planning and implementing health initiatives, including organizing health camps and distributing health-related resources.

Outcome: Through the community-based participatory approach, the women in the village became more aware of their health needs and rights. Maternal and infant mortality rates decreased significantly as more women accessed prenatal care and safe delivery services. The village's Women's Health Committee continues to lead health initiatives, making sustainable changes in women's health and well-being.

Case Study 6: *Youth-Led Mental Health Initiative in an Urban Slum in Country Y*

Context: In an urban slum in Country Y, the prevalence of mental health issues among youth was on the rise, exacerbated by poverty, violence, and limited access to mental health services. A community-based participatory approach was adopted to address the mental health needs of the youth in the community.

Key Components of the Community-Based Participatory Approach:

- Youth Participation: Local youth were actively involved in the planning and design of the mental health initiative. They shared their experiences, concerns, and aspirations, ensuring that the intervention was relevant and engaging for their age group.
- Partnership with Mental Health Professionals: The community partnered with mental health professionals and organizations to provide training and guidance to youth facilitators. This built the capacity of the youth to support their peers dealing with mental health challenges.
- Safe Spaces: The community created safe spaces within the slum where youth could freely express themselves, seek support, and engage in mental health awareness activities.
- Stigma Reduction: The initiative focused on reducing the stigma associated with mental health issues. Youth-led campaigns and awareness sessions were conducted to educate the community about mental health and promote empathy and understanding.

Outcome: The youth-led mental health initiative had a transformative impact on the community. Youth facilitators developed strong leadership and counseling skills, providing crucial mental health support to their peers. As stigma reduced, more youth sought help, and mental health awareness became an integral part of community discussions. The initiative became a model for other communities facing similar mental health challenges, promoting the value of youth engagement in mental health advocacy.

Conclusion: These case studies illustrate the power of the community-based participatory approach in addressing diverse health challenges in different contexts. By involving community members, fostering partnerships, and empowering individuals to take charge of their health, community-based participatory approaches lead to transformative changes that are sustainable and tailored to the unique needs of each community. These case studies exemplify the potential of collaborative efforts in building resilient communities and promoting equitable health outcomes.

CONCLUSION

Community-based participatory approaches offer a transformative framework for public health interventions in developing nations. By engaging communities, promoting inclusivity and equity, and strengthening partnerships with stakeholders, public health professionals can create interventions that are contextually relevant, sustainable, and equitable. Embracing the principles of community participation and collaboration, these approaches pave the way for healthier and more resilient communities where everyone has a voice and access to essential health services.

REFERENCES

[1]   Israel BA, Schulz AJ, Parker EA, Becker AB. Review of community-based research: assessing partnership approaches to improve public health. Annu Rev Public Health 1998; 19(1): 173-202.
[http://dx.doi.org/10.1146/annurev.publhealth.19.1.173] [PMID: 9611617]

[2]   Wallerstein NB, Duran B. Using community-based participatory research to address health disparities. Health Promot Pract 2006; 7(3): 312-23.
[http://dx.doi.org/10.1177/1524839906289376] [PMID: 16760238]

[3]   Minkler M, Wallerstein N, Eds. Community-Based Participatory Research for Health: From Process to Outcomes. 2nd ed., John Wiley & Sons 2008.

[4]   Jones L, Wells K. Strategies for academic and clinician engagement in community-participatory partnered research. JAMA 2007; 297(4): 407-10.
[http://dx.doi.org/10.1001/jama.297.4.407] [PMID: 17244838]

[5]   Cargo M, Mercer SL. The value and challenges of participatory research: strengthening its practice. Annu Rev Public Health 2008; 29(1): 325-50.
[http://dx.doi.org/10.1146/annurev.publhealth.29.091307.083824] [PMID: 18173388]

[6]   Viswanathan M, Ammerman A, Eng E, *et al.* Community-based participatory research: Assessing the evidence: Summary. Rockville, MD: Agency for Healthcare Research and Quality 2004. Available from: https://www.ncbi.nlm.nih.gov/books/NBK11852/

CHAPTER 5

Addressing Communicable Diseases

Abstract: Communicable diseases remain a significant public health challenge in developing nations, impacting communities' health and resilience. This chapter explores strategies for preventing and controlling infectious diseases, including health education, sanitation, vector control, and sustainable interventions. Additionally, it discusses the importance of immunization campaigns, disease surveillance, and managing outbreaks and pandemics in resource-limited settings. By implementing comprehensive and community-centered approaches, developing nations can enhance their resilience and mitigate the burden of communicable diseases.

Keywords: Communicable diseases, Control, Disease surveillance, Immunization campaigns, Outbreaks, Pandemics, Prevention, Resource-limited settings.

INTRODUCTION

Infectious diseases pose significant challenges to public health in developing nations. This section outlines key strategies for preventing and controlling these diseases, focusing on health education, sanitation, vector control, and sustainable interventions. By empowering communities and strengthening healthcare systems, these strategies contribute to building resilience and improving public health outcomes.

Immunization campaigns and disease surveillance are vital components of public health strategies to combat communicable diseases. This section discusses the importance of immunization campaigns in reaching vulnerable populations and addressing vaccine hesitancy. It also highlights the role of disease surveillance in early detection and response to outbreaks, emphasizing the need for strong community engagement and international collaboration.

Managing outbreaks and pandemics in resource-limited settings requires coordinated efforts and effective response strategies. This section explores the challenges and strategies in responding to outbreaks, including establishing rapid response teams, enhancing healthcare systems, and leveraging international collaboration. By prioritizing preparedness and resilience-building measures, developing nations can mitigate the impact of communicable diseases on public health.

Strategies for Preventing and Controlling Infectious Diseases

Infectious diseases continue to be a significant burden on public health, particularly in developing nations. Preventing and controlling these diseases requires a comprehensive and integrated approach that involves individuals, communities, healthcare systems, and public health authorities. This section will delve into critical strategies for preventing and controlling infectious diseases in developing communities, focusing on health education, sanitation, vector control, and sustainable interventions to build resilience and improve public health outcomes [1, 2].

Health Education and Awareness

Health education is a fundamental strategy for preventing and controlling infectious diseases. By increasing awareness and knowledge about disease transmission, symptoms, and preventive measures, communities can be better equipped to protect themselves and respond effectively. Local healthcare workers, community leaders, and public health professionals are crucial in disseminating information through various channels such as workshops, community meetings, radio programs, and educational materials.

Community-based health education initiatives are particularly effective as they are tailored to the community's specific cultural and social context. Engaging with community members in their native language and understanding local beliefs and practices can foster trust and improve the acceptance of preventive measures. These educational efforts can address many diseases, including waterborne diseases, vector-borne diseases, respiratory infections, and sexually transmitted infections.

Sanitation and Hygiene

Access to clean water and proper sanitation facilities is fundamental to preventing waterborne diseases and gastrointestinal infections. In resource-limited settings, inadequate sanitation infrastructure poses a significant public health challenge. Encouraging the use of latrines, promoting handwashing with soap, and ensuring safe drinking water sources can significantly reduce the transmission of infectious agents.

Sanitation and hygiene interventions can be integrated into community development projects, focusing on sustainable practices to ensure long-term benefits. Community members' active participation in the planning and implementation of sanitation initiatives can enhance the ownership and maintenance of facilities.

Vector Control

Vector-borne diseases, such as malaria, dengue fever, and Zika virus, are a significant health concern in many developing nations. Vector control strategies aim to reduce the population of disease-carrying vectors and disrupt their transmission cycle. Insecticide-treated bed nets, indoor residual spraying, and environmental management to eliminate breeding sites are among the effective vector control measures.

Community involvement in vector control is essential to its success. Engaging community members in identifying breeding sites and implementing control measures fosters a sense of ownership and responsibility for disease prevention. Furthermore, collaboration with local environmental and agricultural authorities can strengthen vector control efforts by promoting safe and eco-friendly practices.

Sustainable Interventions

Sustainability is critical when implementing interventions to prevent and control infectious diseases in developing communities. One-time interventions may offer short-term benefits, but sustainable approaches that integrate into existing healthcare systems are more likely to yield long-lasting results.

Building local capacity through training healthcare workers, equipping health facilities with necessary resources, and improving disease surveillance systems contribute to the resilience of communities in combating infectious diseases. Collaborating with international organizations and donor agencies can help secure funding and technical expertise for sustainable public health programs.

Conclusion: Strategies for preventing and controlling infectious diseases in developing nations require a multi-pronged approach addressing various community health aspects. Health education, sanitation, vector control, and sustainable interventions are vital components that contribute to building resilient communities capable of navigating public health challenges effectively. By empowering individuals, engaging communities, and strengthening healthcare systems, developing nations can make significant progress in curbing the burden of infectious diseases and promoting overall public health and well-being.

Immunization Campaigns and Disease Surveillance

Immunization campaigns and disease surveillance are vital components of public health strategies in developing nations to prevent and control communicable diseases. These interventions play a critical role in reducing the burden of infectious diseases, protecting vulnerable populations, and ensuring early detection and response to outbreaks. In this section, we will explore the significance of immunization campaigns and disease surveillance, their implementation challenges, and how they contribute to building resilient communities in the face of public health challenges [3 - 5].

Immunization Campaigns

Immunization campaigns are targeted efforts to vaccinate communities, especially those at risk, against vaccine-preventable diseases. Vaccines are one of the most cost-effective public health interventions, preventing millions of deaths worldwide. In developing nations, where access to healthcare may be limited, immunization campaigns play a crucial role in reaching remote and underserved populations.

- *Vaccine Access and Distribution:* Challenges in delivering vaccines to remote and resource-limited areas necessitate innovative approaches. Mobile vaccination teams, community outreach programs, and collaboration with local healthcare providers facilitate vaccine distribution and accessibility. Public-private partnerships and support from international organizations can also strengthen the availability of vaccines.
- *Addressing Vaccine Hesitancy:* Vaccine hesitancy, fueled by misinformation and distrust, poses challenges to successful immunization campaigns. Culturally tailored health education and community engagement efforts are essential to address concerns and build trust in vaccines. Engaging community influencers, religious leaders, and healthcare workers as vaccine advocates can increase acceptance and uptake.
- *Targeting High-Risk Groups:* Immunization campaigns often prioritize high-risk groups, such as infants, pregnant women, and the elderly. Ensuring vaccination coverage in these populations is crucial to protect vulnerable individuals and prevent disease outbreaks.

Disease Surveillance

Disease surveillance involves systematically monitoring, collecting, analyzing, and interpreting health data to detect and respond to infectious disease threats. It serves as an early warning system, enabling prompt public health interventions to prevent outbreaks from spreading.

- *Early Detection of Outbreaks:* Effective disease surveillance enables the early detection of infectious disease outbreaks. By monitoring patterns of illness and identifying unusual trends, public health authorities can take swift action to contain and control the spread of diseases.
- *Strengthening Laboratory Capacity:* A robust laboratory network is essential for accurate disease diagnosis and identification. Investing in laboratory infrastructure, equipment, and training for healthcare personnel strengthens disease surveillance capabilities in resource-limited settings.
- *Integrated Disease Surveillance and Response Systems:* Integrating disease surveillance systems with existing health information systems and technology enhances data sharing, analysis, and reporting. This integration improves the timeliness and quality of surveillance data, enabling real-time decision-making.

Conclusion: Immunization campaigns and disease surveillance are critical pillars in the fight against communicable diseases in developing nations. Immunization campaigns protect populations from vaccine-preventable diseases and ensure equity in accessing life-saving vaccines. Disease surveillance, on the other hand, enables early detection of outbreaks and prompt response, preventing further transmission and saving lives.

Both interventions require strong community engagement, investment in healthcare infrastructure, and collaboration among various stakeholders, including governments, international organizations, non-governmental organizations, and local communities. By implementing effective immunization campaigns and robust disease surveillance systems, developing nations can bolster their resilience against infectious diseases, promote public health, and achieve sustainable development goals.

Managing Outbreaks and Pandemics in Resource-Limited Settings

Outbreaks of infectious diseases and pandemics can have devastating effects on communities, particularly in resource-limited settings. The management of such crises requires prompt and effective responses to prevent further transmission, provide adequate healthcare, and mitigate the impact on public health. This section will explore the challenges and strategies in managing outbreaks and pandemics in resource-limited settings, focusing on building resilience through community engagement, healthcare preparedness, and international collaboration [6, 7].

Rapid Response Teams and Community Engagement

In resource-limited settings, establishing rapid response teams is crucial for effectively managing outbreaks. These multidisciplinary teams, including healthcare professionals, epidemiologists, and community health workers, can respond swiftly to identify cases, conduct contact tracing, and implement necessary public health measures.

Community engagement is equally vital during outbreaks and pandemics. Transparent communication about the situation, preventive measures, and available healthcare services fosters trust and cooperation within the community. Local leaders, community influencers, and traditional healers are vital in disseminating accurate information and encouraging compliance with public health guidelines.

Isolation and Quarantine Facilities

Isolation and quarantine facilities are essential for controlling the spread of infectious diseases during outbreaks. In resource-limited settings, creating and maintaining such facilities can be challenging due to limited healthcare infrastructure. However, repurposing existing facilities, setting up temporary medical tents, and partnering with community centers can provide effective solutions.

Providing adequate care and support to individuals in isolation or quarantine is vital. Ensuring access to medical treatment, mental health support, and essential supplies will not only improve patient outcomes but also encourage voluntary compliance with public health measures.

Strengthening Healthcare Systems

Healthcare systems in resource-limited settings often face significant strain during outbreaks and pandemics. Building resilience in these settings involves strengthening healthcare infrastructure, training healthcare personnel, and ensuring adequate supply chains for medical equipment and medications.

Investments in telemedicine and digital health solutions can also enhance healthcare delivery during crises. Telemedicine platforms enable remote consultations, disease monitoring, and the dissemination of health information, thereby alleviating the burden on healthcare facilities and reducing the risk of transmission.

International Collaboration and Aid

Managing outbreaks and pandemics in resource-limited settings often requires international collaboration and aid. International organizations, donor agencies, and foreign governments can provide critical support in terms of funding, technical expertise, and medical supplies.

Coordination among global health partners is essential to avoid duplication of efforts and ensure a cohesive response. International collaboration can also facilitate the exchange of best practices, lessons learned, and the deployment of medical personnel to areas experiencing high caseloads.

In conclusion, managing outbreaks and pandemics in resource-limited settings demands a comprehensive and collaborative approach. Rapid response teams, community engagement, and isolation facilities are key components of an effective response. Strengthening healthcare systems and leveraging technology are crucial for providing adequate care and support during crises. International collaboration and aid are essential to support resource-limited settings in their response efforts. By building resilience through proactive preparedness, robust healthcare systems, and international solidarity, developing nations can navigate the challenges posed by outbreaks and pandemics, protect public health, and strengthen their capacity to address future public health challenges.

Case Study 7: *Strategies for Preventing and Controlling Infectious Diseases.*

This case study looks at 'Combating Malaria in Sub-Saharan Africa - The Roll Back Malaria Initiative.'

Introduction: Malaria remains a significant public health challenge, particularly in sub-Saharan Africa, where the burden of the disease is most severe. To combat this infectious disease, the Roll Back Malaria (RBM) initiative was launched as a global partnership in 1998. The initiative aimed to strengthen prevention and control measures, reduce malaria-related deaths, and eventually eliminate malaria in the region.

Background: Sub-Saharan Africa accounts for over 90% of global malaria cases and deaths, affecting vulnerable populations, including pregnant women and young children. The RBM initiative recognized the need for a multi-pronged approach to address malaria comprehensively.

Implementation: The RBM initiative adopted several strategies for preventing and controlling malaria:

1. Vector Control: Emphasizing the use of insecticide-treated bed nets (ITNs) to protect individuals from mosquito bites, particularly during sleep, as well as indoor residual spraying to reduce mosquito populations.

2. Early Diagnosis and Treatment: Increasing access to rapid diagnostic tests (RDTs) to diagnose malaria promptly and ensuring the availability of effective antimalarial medications for prompt treatment.

3. Health Education and Community Engagement: Conducting health education campaigns to raise awareness about malaria prevention and control measures, promoting the proper use of ITNs, and engaging communities in malaria control efforts.

4. Surveillance and Data Analysis: Establishing robust surveillance systems to track malaria cases, monitor drug resistance, and evaluate the impact of intervention strategies.

Results: The RBM initiative's concerted efforts have shown promising results in the fight against malaria in sub-Saharan Africa. Between 2000 and 2019, malaria-related deaths declined by 44% in the region, with substantial progress made in increasing ITN coverage and access to malaria diagnosis and treatment. However, challenges remain, and ongoing commitment is required to sustain the gains and eliminate malaria entirely.

Case Study 8: *Immunization Campaigns and Disease Surveillance during the Ebola Outbreak in West Africa.*

This case study looks at 'Strengthening Health Systems to Control Ebola Virus Disease.'

Introduction: The Ebola virus disease (EVD) outbreak that struck West Africa in 2014-2016 highlighted the critical importance of robust immunization campaigns and disease surveillance systems in resource-limited settings. The outbreak presented significant challenges in detecting and containing the disease, but valuable lessons were learned to improve future responses.

Background: The EVD outbreak in West Africa was the largest and most complex Ebola outbreak in history. Guinea, Sierra Leone, and Liberia were the hardest-hit countries, facing unprecedented challenges in controlling the spread of the virus due to weak health systems and limited resources.

Implementation: During the Ebola outbreak, several strategies were employed to strengthen disease surveillance and control measures:

- Immunization Campaigns: The deployment of experimental Ebola vaccines, such as rVSV-ZEBOV-GP, in affected regions played a crucial role in curbing the outbreak. Large-scale vaccination campaigns targeted high-risk individuals, including healthcare workers and contacts of confirmed cases.
- Contact Tracing: Robust contact tracing efforts were implemented to identify and monitor individuals who had been in contact with Ebola-infected patients, facilitating prompt isolation and treatment.

- Training and Capacity Building: Health workers and community volunteers were trained in infection prevention and control measures, safe burials, and other aspects of EVD management.
- Cross-Border Collaboration: Regional collaboration and information sharing were essential for coordinating response efforts across borders.

Results: The timely implementation of immunization campaigns, contact tracing, and other control measures helped contain the Ebola outbreak in West Africa. While the outbreak led to significant loss of life and immense suffering, the experience provided valuable insights into the importance of preparedness, early detection, and community engagement in managing infectious disease outbreaks.

Conclusion: These case studies exemplify the critical role of proactive strategies for preventing and controlling infectious diseases in resource-limited settings. By implementing immunization campaigns, enhancing disease surveillance, and fostering community engagement, public health systems can effectively manage outbreaks and pandemics, leading to better health outcomes for communities in developing nations. These lessons must be integrated into ongoing efforts to build resilient health systems that can respond effectively to current and future public health challenges.

CONCLUSION

Addressing communicable diseases in developing nations requires a multifaceted approach that integrates community engagement, healthcare infrastructure strengthening, and international collaboration. By implementing comprehensive strategies for prevention, control, and outbreak management, developing nations can improve public health outcomes, enhance resilience, and mitigate the burden of communicable diseases on communities. Embracing a proactive and collaborative approach is essential for building healthier and more resilient societies.

REFERENCES

[1]   World Health Organization. Preventing disease through healthy environments: A global assessment of the burden of disease from environmental risks. World Health Organization, 2019. Available from: https://www.who.int/publications/i/item/9789241565196

[2]   United Nations International Children's Emergency Fund (UNICEF). Malaria - Prevention and Control. UNICEF, 2021. Available from: https://data.unicef.org/topic/child-health/malaria/

[3]   World Health Organization. Global Vaccine Action Plan 2011-2020. World Health Organization, 2021. Available from: https://www.who.int/immunization/global_vaccine_action_plan/GVAP_doc_2011_2020/en/

[4]   Thacker SB, Stroup DF, Moolenaar RL. Epidemiology and public health surveillance. In: Detels BS, Beaglehole R, Lansang MA, Gulliford M, Eds. Oxford Textbook of Public Health. 3rd ed. Oxford University Press 1996; pp. 140-58.

[5]   Saleh J. Concise Handbook of Epidemiology. 1st ed., Amazon Books 2017.

[6]   Heymann DL, Chen L, Takemi K, *et al.* Global health security: the wider lessons from the west African Ebola virus disease epidemic. Lancet 2015; 385(9980): 1884-901.
[http://dx.doi.org/10.1016/S0140-6736(15)60858-3] [PMID: 25987157]

[7]   J Olumade T, A Adesanya O, J Fred-Akintunwa I, *et al.* Infectious disease outbreak preparedness and response in Nigeria: history, limitations and recommendations for global health policy and practice. AIMS Public Health 2020; 7(4): 736-57.
[http://dx.doi.org/10.3934/publichealth.2020057] [PMID: 33294478]

CHAPTER 6

Non-Communicable Diseases and Lifestyle Interventions

Abstract: Non-communicable diseases (NCDs) pose a significant public health challenge in developing nations, with chronic conditions such as cardiovascular diseases, diabetes, cancer, and respiratory illnesses contributing to a substantial burden of morbidity and mortality. This chapter explores the rise of NCDs, emphasizing the importance of promoting healthy behaviors and lifestyle changes, as well as improving access to healthcare for effective NCD management. Understanding the multifaceted reasons behind the rise of NCDs and implementing comprehensive strategies can mitigate this growing public health concern and foster resilience within communities.

Keywords: Developing nations, Healthy behaviours, Healthcare access, Lifestyle interventions, Non-communicable diseases, NCDs.

INTRODUCTION

Non-communicable diseases (NCDs) have become a leading cause of morbidity and mortality worldwide, with developing nations experiencing a significant increase in their prevalence. This section explores the reasons behind the rise of NCDs, including demographic transitions, urbanization, changes in dietary habits, and limited access to healthcare. Addressing these challenges requires a comprehensive approach that focuses on prevention, early detection, and effective management of NCDs. By unraveling the complex factors contributing to the rise of NCDs, communities and public health practitioners can design targeted interventions to mitigate this growing public health concern.

Promoting healthy behaviors and lifestyle changes is essential in preventing and managing NCDs. This section discusses strategies for raising awareness about the risks of unhealthy behaviors, encouraging physical activity, improving dietary habits, and implementing policies to control tobacco and alcohol use. By empowering individuals with knowledge, fostering community collaboration, and creating environments that support healthier choices, communities can effectively address the rising burden of NCDs and improve overall well-being.

Effective management of NCDs requires improving access to healthcare services in resource-limited settings. This section explores strategies for strengthening primary healthcare systems, training healthcare providers, and leveraging technology to expand access to NCD care. Task-shifting, community health worker programs, telemedicine, and integrated NCD clinics are essential components of efforts to improve healthcare access and enhance NCD management. By implementing comprehensive lifestyle interventions and enhancing healthcare systems, developing nations can effectively combat the rise of NCDs and improve population health outcomes.

Understanding the Rise of Non-Communicable Diseases

In recent decades, a significant shift in disease burden has occurred, with non-communicable diseases (NCDs) taking center stage as the leading causes of morbidity and mortality worldwide. NCDs encompass various chronic health conditions, such as cardiovascular diseases, diabetes, cancers, and chronic respiratory diseases. While traditionally associated with affluent societies, the prevalence of NCDs has been rapidly rising in developing nations [1].

The rise of NCDs can be attributed to various factors, including demographic transitions, urbanization, and changes in dietary habits and physical activity levels. In developing nations, rapid urbanization and shifts in lifestyle patterns have led to an increased prevalence of risk factors such as sedentary behavior, unhealthy diets, tobacco use, and excessive alcohol consumption [1, 2].

Economic development and globalization have also influenced the rise of NCDs by promoting the consumption of processed foods, sugary beverages, and tobacco products. Additionally, limited access to healthcare and health education in many developing communities further exacerbates the burden of NCDs. Addressing these challenges requires a comprehensive approach that combines prevention, early detection, and effective management of NCDs. Public health efforts must focus on promoting healthy behaviors, advocating for lifestyle changes, and enhancing healthcare systems to provide adequate support for NCD management [1, 2].

This section seeks to unravel the multifaceted reasons behind this rise and emphasizes the crucial role of lifestyle interventions in addressing this public health challenge.

- *Epidemiological Transition:* The epidemiological transition describes the shift from a predominance of infectious diseases to NCDs as the primary health concern in a population. Developing nations are currently undergoing this transition, often facing a dual burden of infectious diseases and NCDs. Factors contributing to this transition include urbanization, changes in diet, reduced physical activity, and an aging population. The interaction of these factors results in a complex interplay that accelerates the prevalence of NCDs.

- *Lifestyle Changes:* Urbanization, as a hallmark of development, often leads to changes in lifestyle and behaviors. The adoption of sedentary lifestyles, characterized by increased screen time, desk-bound jobs, and reduced physical activity, contributes to obesity, cardiovascular diseases, and diabetes. Additionally, dietary shifts towards energy-dense, nutrient-poor foods high in sugar, salt, and unhealthy fats further exacerbate NCD prevalence.
- *Socioeconomic Determinants:* Socioeconomic factors play a pivotal role in the rise of NCDs. Poverty and limited access to education can lead to poor health literacy and limited awareness of healthy lifestyle choices. Inadequate healthcare systems may result in late diagnosis and suboptimal management of NCDs. Furthermore, disparities in access to nutritious foods and recreational spaces amplify the burden of NCDs among marginalized populations.
- *Globalization and Cultural Influences:* Globalization has facilitated the spread of Western dietary patterns and sedentary lifestyles to developing nations. Traditional diets rich in whole grains, vegetables, and fruits have been replaced with processed foods, contributing to obesity and its associated NCDs. Cultural beliefs and practices may also hinder the adoption of healthier lifestyles, necessitating culturally sensitive interventions.
- *Tobacco and Alcohol Use:* Tobacco use and excessive alcohol consumption are significant risk factors for NCDs, including lung cancer, cardiovascular diseases, and liver diseases. Developing nations often face challenges in implementing effective tobacco and alcohol control policies, allowing these risk factors to contribute to the rise of NCDs.

Conclusion: By understanding the intricate factors fueling the rise of NCDs, communities and public health practitioners can design tailored interventions that promote healthier lifestyles, foster community engagement, and ultimately contribute to mitigating this growing public health concern. The rise of non-communicable diseases in developing nations is a multifaceted phenomenon driven by the interplay of urbanization, lifestyle changes, socioeconomic factors, globalization, and cultural influences. Addressing this challenge requires a comprehensive approach integrating health education, policy changes, and community-based interventions. Empowering communities to make healthier lifestyle choices, improving access to healthcare, and implementing regulations to control tobacco and alcohol use are pivotal steps toward building resilient communities capable of navigating the complex landscape of non-communicable diseases [1, 2].

Promoting Healthy Behaviours and Lifestyle Changes

In the face of the rising burden of non-communicable diseases (NCDs) in developing nations, promoting healthy behaviors and encouraging lifestyle changes have become paramount. Promoting healthy behaviors and lifestyle changes is crucial in preventing and managing NCDs. Health education campaigns can raise awareness about the risks of unhealthy behaviors and the benefits of adopting healthier choices. Engaging individuals and communities through workshops, media campaigns, and school-based interventions can foster a culture of health and well-being [3].

Encouraging regular physical activity is paramount in NCD prevention. Promoting active transportation, creating safe spaces for exercise, and incorporating physical education in schools can help combat sedentary behavior. Likewise, addressing dietary habits involves promoting the consumption of fresh fruits, vegetables, and whole grains while reducing the intake of processed and unhealthy foods [3, 4].

Tobacco use and excessive alcohol consumption are significant risk factors for NCDs. Implementing tobacco control policies, such as higher taxes on tobacco products and smoke-free public spaces, can curb smoking rates. Similarly, measures like alcohol taxation and restrictions on alcohol advertising can help reduce alcohol-related harm [3, 4].

This section explores the multifaceted strategies that can be harnessed to facilitate the adoption of healthier habits within communities, thereby mitigating the impact of NCDs and fostering resilience.

- *Health Education and Awareness:* Effective health education campaigns serve as the cornerstone of promoting healthy behaviors. Tailored messaging that emphasizes the risks associated with unhealthy lifestyles, such as smoking, excessive alcohol consumption, poor diet, and lack of physical activity, can empower individuals to make informed decisions about their health. Utilizing culturally sensitive communication channels, such as community gatherings, radio broadcasts, and local influencers, enhances the reach and impact of such campaigns.
- *Community Engagement:* Engaging communities in designing and implementing health interventions foster a sense of ownership and increases the likelihood of sustained behavior change. Community-based workshops, support groups, and peer-led initiatives can provide a platform for sharing experiences, setting collective goals, and holding each other accountable for lifestyle modifications.
- *Infrastructure and Accessibility:* Creating environments that facilitate healthier choices is crucial. Developing safe and accessible recreational spaces,

pedestrian-friendly pathways, and public transportation options can encourage physical activity. Likewise, ensuring the availability and affordability of fresh, nutritious foods through farmers' markets, community gardens, and urban planning strategies supports dietary improvements.

- *Policy Interventions:* Policy changes can have a significant impact on shaping individual behaviors. Implementing measures such as taxation on tobacco products and sugary beverages, restrictions on marketing unhealthy foods to children, and mandating clear nutritional labeling empowers consumers to make healthier choices and reduces exposure to risk factors.
- *Workplace Wellness Programs:* Given the substantial amount of time individuals spend at work, implementing workplace wellness programs can have a positive influence on behavior change. Offering incentives for physical activity, promoting healthy cafeteria options, and providing resources for stress management can create a supportive environment for employees to adopt healthier lifestyles.
- *School-Based Initiatives:* Schools play a vital role in shaping children's habits and knowledge. Integrating health education into the curriculum, offering nutritious meals, and providing opportunities for physical activity during school hours contribute to establishing a foundation of healthy behaviors from a young age.
- *Behavioral Economics and Nudges:* Behavioural economics principles, such as nudges, can guide individuals towards healthier choices without restricting their autonomy. For instance, placing fruits at eye level in grocery stores or sending personalized text reminders for physical activity can gently steer behavior in the desired direction.

Conclusion: Promoting healthy behaviors and lifestyle changes within developing nations requires a multi-pronged approach that spans education, community engagement, infrastructure development, policy reform, workplace initiatives, and innovative behavioral techniques. By empowering individuals with knowledge, fostering community collaboration, and creating environments that support healthier choices, communities can effectively navigate the challenges posed by non-communicable diseases. Ultimately, cultivating resilient communities hinges on their ability to adapt and embrace healthier lifestyles, leading to improved overall well-being and reduced NCD prevalence [3, 4].

Expanding the Role of Resilient Communities in NCD Management

Community-based interventions are critical in addressing NCDs, particularly in resource-constrained settings. Resilient communities can act as the backbone of sustainable interventions, using local knowledge, social capital, and collective action to tackle NCDs effectively. By fostering resilience, communities can adapt to the challenges posed by urbanization, lifestyle changes, and socioeconomic factors [5, 6].

Framework for Community-Based NCD Interventions

1. Community-Led Health Promotion Programs: Engaging local leaders and health advocates in designing and implementing health promotion activities ensures that interventions are culturally relevant and accepted. For example, in rural areas, local leaders such as village elders or religious leaders can champion lifestyle changes like promoting healthy diets and regular physical activity. Communities can organize local health days focused on educating residents about healthy food choices and the risks associated with tobacco, alcohol, and sedentary lifestyles.

2. Participatory Action Planning: Communities should be directly involved in identifying their own NCD risks and co-creating interventions. Using participatory approaches such as community forums and workshops allows for open dialogue on local health concerns. For instance, a participatory rural appraisal (PRA) can be used to map areas with poor access to healthcare and unhealthy food options, identifying barriers to NCD management. In this process, communities can identify feasible solutions like establishing walking groups for physical activity or organizing group purchases of fresh produce from nearby farmers.

3. Community Health Worker (CHW) Programs: CHWs play a pivotal role in extending NCD care to underserved populations. They can provide health education, monitor patients' conditions, and support adherence to treatment protocols. By building capacity within the community, CHWs empower individuals to take control of their health and create lasting change. A successful example would be training CHWs to monitor blood pressure and glucose levels, offering early detection and management of hypertension and diabetes at the community level.

4. Collective Monitoring and Feedback Mechanisms: Communities can establish their systems to monitor health outcomes and provide continuous feedback on interventions. For example, digital platforms where community members report their health status or challenges they face in accessing services can allow for real-time adjustments to interventions. This continuous feedback loop strengthens the resilience of the community by ensuring interventions are adaptive and responsive to changing needs.

5. Resilient Community Networks for Support: Peer-support networks can be established within communities to help individuals manage NCDs. These

networks provide emotional and practical support, reinforcing lifestyle changes and fostering accountability. For instance, groups of people with diabetes can meet regularly to discuss their progress in managing their condition, share dietary tips, and encourage one another to stay active.

Examples

- Rural Hypertension Monitoring Program: In rural areas with limited access to healthcare, community health workers can lead weekly blood pressure monitoring sessions at local community centers. The data collected can help healthcare providers prioritize patients who need urgent care. The community members can also be trained to recognize the signs of hypertension and refer at-risk individuals to healthcare providers.
- Urban Youth-Led NCD Awareness Campaigns: In urban settings, youth can lead campaigns to promote physical activity and healthy eating. They can organize community events like street football matches, cooking classes focusing on local, healthy recipes, and competitions to reduce tobacco and alcohol consumption. These activities empower youth to be active participants in reducing NCD risks in their communities.

Improving Access to Healthcare for NCD Management

Effective management of NCDs requires improving access to healthcare services in resource-limited settings. Strengthening primary healthcare systems, training healthcare providers, and increasing the availability of essential medicines are essential steps in enhancing NCD management [7]. Task-shifting and community health worker programs can improve access to NCD care, particularly in underserved areas. These programs empower community health workers to screen for NCD risk factors, provide health education, and support patients in adhering to treatment plans. Integrating NCD care into existing healthcare services can improve efficiency and reduce the burden on specialized facilities. Telemedicine and mobile health applications can also expand access to healthcare, particularly in remote regions, by enabling remote consultations and patient monitoring [7, 8].

Access to quality healthcare services is a cornerstone in addressing the escalating burden of NCDs in developing nations. This section explores the critical role of accessible healthcare in managing NCDs. It provides insights into strategies that can be employed to ensure that individuals and communities have the necessary resources to prevent, diagnose, and manage these chronic conditions effectively [7, 8].

- *Primary Care Strengthening:* Strengthening primary healthcare services is essential for NCD management. This involves training healthcare providers in identifying and managing NCDs and establishing clinics that offer comprehensive services related to prevention, early detection, treatment, and follow-up. These clinics can serve as the first point of contact for individuals seeking care, enabling timely interventions.

- *Task Shifting and Training:* Given the shortage of specialized healthcare professionals in many developing nations, task shifting involves training non-specialized healthcare workers, such as community health workers and nurses, to provide basic NCD-related services. This approach not only enhances accessibility but also optimizes the existing workforce.
- *Telemedicine and Mobile Health (mHealth):* Leveraging technology, including telemedicine and mobile health applications, can bridge geographical barriers and improve access to healthcare services. Teleconsultations, remote monitoring, and health education through mobile apps can provide individuals with expert guidance and support, particularly in remote or underserved areas.
- *Integrated NCD Clinics:* Creating specialized clinics or centers dedicated to NCD management can streamline care delivery. These clinics can offer a range of services, from screenings and diagnosis to counseling, treatment, and rehabilitation. By consolidating resources, these centers ensure comprehensive and coordinated care.
- *Medications and Supplies Availability:* Ensuring a consistent supply of essential medications and medical supplies is crucial for NCD management. Collaborations with pharmaceutical companies, government agencies, and international organizations can help address the challenges of affordability, availability, and quality of medications.

In conclusion, non-communicable diseases are a growing public health concern in developing nations, driven by changes in lifestyle, urbanization, and economic development. Promoting healthy behaviors and lifestyle changes is crucial to address the rise of NCDs. Health education, physical activity promotion, tobacco control, and alcohol regulation are integral to preventive efforts. Improving access to healthcare and strengthening primary healthcare systems are essential for effective NCD management. Task-shifting and community health worker programs can extend NCD care to underserved communities. Integrating NCD services into existing healthcare settings and leveraging digital health solutions can further enhance access to care. By implementing comprehensive lifestyle interventions and enhancing healthcare systems, developing nations can effectively combat the rise of NCDs and improve their populations' overall health and well-being [7, 8].

Case Study 9: This case study examines 'A Workplace Wellness Program in Country X - Promoting Healthy Lifestyles.'

Introduction: Workplace wellness programs are effective platforms for promoting healthy behaviors and lifestyle changes among employees. In country X, a large manufacturing company implemented a workplace wellness program to address the rising prevalence of NCDs among its workforce.

Implementation: The workplace wellness program included the following components:

1. Health Education: Regular health education sessions were conducted to raise awareness about NCD risk factors, healthy eating, physical activity, and stress management.

2. Physical Activity Initiatives: The company provided on-site fitness facilities and organized group exercise classes during lunch breaks and after working hours.

3. Nutritious Food Options: The company introduced healthier food options in the cafeteria, promoting balanced meals and reducing the availability of unhealthy snacks.

4. Smoking Cessation Support: Smoking cessation programs and resources were made available to employees to support those interested in quitting tobacco use.

Case Study 10: This examines 'Mobile Clinics for NCD Management in Rural Country Z.'

Introduction: In rural areas of Country Z, limited access to healthcare facilities and services poses significant challenges for managing NCDs. To address this issue, a mobile healthcare clinic initiative was implemented to improve access to NCD management services in underserved communities.

Implementation: The mobile clinic initiative involved the following strategies:

1. Mobile Clinics: Equipped with medical equipment and staffed by healthcare professionals, mobile clinics traveled to remote villages and communities on a regular schedule.

2. NCD Screening and Management: The mobile clinics offered NCD screening services, including blood pressure measurements, blood glucose tests, and BMI assessments. Those diagnosed with NCDs were provided with treatment, medication, and counseling.

3. Health Education: Community health workers conducted health education sessions in villages, focusing on NCD prevention, self-management, and the importance of regular check-ups.

4. Referral Services: For more complex cases, the mobile clinic served as a gateway to higher-level healthcare facilities, ensuring continuity of care for patients.

Conclusion: These case studies highlight the importance of understanding the rise of non-communicable diseases, promoting healthy behaviors and lifestyle changes, and improving access to healthcare for NCD management. By implementing targeted interventions, such as workplace wellness programs and mobile clinics, public health systems can effectively address the growing burden of NCDs in both urban and rural settings. Emphasizing prevention, education, and equity-focused approaches is essential for building resilient communities and improving the overall health and well-being of populations affected by non-communicable diseases.

CONCLUSION

Non-communicable diseases present a significant public health challenge in developing nations, driven by changes in lifestyle, urbanization, and socioeconomic factors. Promoting healthy behaviors, improving access to healthcare, and implementing policy interventions are crucial steps in addressing the rise of NCDs. By implementing comprehensive strategies that integrate preventive efforts, lifestyle interventions, and healthcare access improvements, developing nations can mitigate the burden of NCDs and improve overall population health and well-being.

REFERENCES

[1]   World Health Organization. Noncommunicable diseases country profiles 2018. World Health Organization, 2018. Available from: https://apps.who.int/iris/handle/10665/274512

[2]   Beaglehole R, Yach D. Globalisation and the prevention and control of non-communicable disease: the neglected chronic diseases of adults. Lancet 2003; 362(9387): 903-8.
       [http://dx.doi.org/10.1016/S0140-6736(03)14335-8] [PMID: 13678979]

[3]   Prochaska JO, Velicer WF. The transtheoretical model of health behavior change. Am J Health Promot 1997; 12(1): 38-48.
       [http://dx.doi.org/10.4278/0890-1171-12.1.38] [PMID: 10170434]

[4]   Spring B, Moller AC, Coons MJ. Multiple health behaviours: overview and implications. J Public Health (Oxf) 2012; 34(Suppl 1): i3-i10.
       [http://dx.doi.org/10.1093/pubmed/fdr111] [PMID: 22363028]

[5]   Ajisegiri, W.S., Abimbola, S., Tesema, A.G., Odusanya, O.O., Peiris, D., & Joshi, R. The organisation of primary health care service delivery for non-communicable diseases in Nigeria: A case-study analysis. PLOS Glob Public Health. 2022; 2(7): e0000566.
       [http://dx.doi.org/10.1371/journal.pgph.0000566] [PMID: 36962373] [PMCID: PMC10021956]

[6]   Hadian, M., Mozafari, M.R., Mazaheri, E., & Jabbari, A. Challenges of the Health System in Preventing Non-Communicable Diseases; Systematized Review. Int J Prev Med. 2021; 12: 71.
       [http://dx.doi.org/10.4103/ijpvm.IJPVM_487_20]

[7]   World Health Organization. Package of Essential Noncommunicable (PEN) Disease Interventions for Primary Health Care. World Health Organization, 2020. Available from: https://www.who.int/publications/i/item/9789240009226

[8]   Geldsetzer P, Manne-Goehler J, Marcus ME, *et al.* The state of hypertension care in 44 low-income and middle-income countries: a cross-sectional study of nationally representative individual-level data from 1·1 million adults. Lancet 2019; 394(10199): 652-62.
[http://dx.doi.org/10.1016/S0140-6736(19)30955-9] [PMID: 31327566]

CHAPTER 7

Comprehensive Care for Mothers and Children

Abstract: Maternal and child health is a cornerstone of public health, especially in developing nations, where ensuring the well-being of women during pregnancy, childbirth, and postpartum, as well as promoting optimal growth and development in children, is crucial. This chapter highlights the significance of enhancing maternal care and safe childbirth practices, implementing childhood immunization and nutrition programs, and preventing and managing common childhood illnesses. By prioritizing these interventions, communities can reduce maternal and infant mortality rates, improve health outcomes, and build resilience. Empowering women, engaging communities, and strengthening healthcare systems are essential for sustained progress in maternal and child health.

Keywords: Childhood illnesses, Community engagement, Child health, Childbirth practices, Immunization, Maternal health, Nutrition programs.

INTRODUCTION

Maternal and child health is a crucial pillar of public health that focuses on ensuring the well-being and survival of women during pregnancy, childbirth, and postpartum, as well as promoting the optimal growth and development of children. Ensuring access to quality maternal care and promoting safe childbirth practices are essential for reducing maternal and infant mortality rates. This section emphasizes the importance of skilled birth attendance, antenatal care, emergency obstetric care, maternal health education, community involvement, birth preparedness, and postnatal care in fostering healthier mothers and thriving infants. By prioritizing these strategies, communities can significantly improve maternal and neonatal outcomes, thus laying the foundation for resilient societies.

Childhood immunization and nutrition programs are critical for preventing infectious diseases and supporting optimal growth and development in children. Vaccines protect children from life-threatening diseases, while proper nutrition during early childhood is essential for their overall well-being. This section explores strategies for ensuring high immunization coverage, promoting exclusive breastfeeding, educating caregivers about proper nutrition, and improving hygiene and sanitation practices. By implementing these interventions, communities can reduce childhood morbidity and mortality rates and promote healthier generations.

Jalal-Eddeen Abubakar Saleh

Preventing and managing common childhood illnesses is vital for reducing child mortality and promoting well-being in developing nations. This section discusses the importance of immunization programs, exclusive breastfeeding, nutrition education, hygiene and sanitation practices, integrated case management, oral rehydration therapy, early recognition of danger signs, community health workers, and incorporating traditional knowledge into healthcare programs. By prioritizing these interventions and engaging communities, societies can effectively prevent and manage childhood illnesses, thus building resilience and improving child health outcomes.

Enhancing Maternal Care and Safe Childbirth Practices

Improving maternal care and ensuring safe childbirth practices are fundamental to reducing maternal mortality and ensuring positive birth outcomes. Prenatal care is a cornerstone of maternal health, providing pregnant women with comprehensive health assessments, screenings, and education. Early detection and management of pregnancy-related complications can significantly improve maternal and neonatal outcomes. Access to skilled birth attendants and emergency obstetric care is essential, especially in resource-limited settings. Encouraging facility-based deliveries with skilled professionals can reduce the risks associated with home births and facilitate timely interventions during childbirth emergencies [1 - 3].

Promoting maternal nutrition and providing essential supplements, such as folic acid and iron, are vital for maternal and fetal health. Additionally, empowering women with knowledge about breastfeeding benefits and providing lactation support contribute to better infant nutrition and early development. The health and well-being of mothers and infants are pivotal for building resilient communities in developing nations. Ensuring access to quality maternal care and promoting safe childbirth practices are paramount in reducing maternal and infant mortality rates. This section delves into the multifaceted strategies that can be employed to enhance maternal care, foster safe childbirth practices, and contribute to healthier mothers and thriving infants [1, 2].

- *Skilled Birth Attendance:* Encouraging skilled birth attendance is a cornerstone of safe childbirth practices. Trained healthcare professionals, such as midwives, nurses, and doctors, are critical in ensuring safe deliveries. Communities should be educated about the benefits of skilled attendants and equipped with the knowledge to seek their services.
- *Antenatal Care:* Early and comprehensive antenatal care is essential for monitoring the health of both the mother and the developing fetus. Regular ant-

enatal visits offer opportunities for health assessments, education about pregnancy and childbirth, and early detection of potential complications.

- *Emergency Obstetric Care:* Establishing access to emergency obstetric care is imperative for managing childbirth complications. This includes timely interventions for hemorrhage, eclampsia, obstructed labor, and other emergencies. Health facilities should have trained staff, essential supplies, and transportation options for rapid referral if needed.
- *Maternal Health Education:* It is crucial to educate expectant mothers and their families about maternal health and safe childbirth practices. Health education sessions can cover topics such as birth preparedness, recognizing danger signs during pregnancy and labor, and understanding the importance of seeking timely care.
- *Community Involvement:* Engaging communities in maternal care and childbirth practices fosters a sense of responsibility and support. Community leaders, local influencers, and women's groups can collaborate with healthcare providers to organize awareness campaigns, workshops, and discussions on maternal health.
- *Birth Preparedness and Complication Readiness:* Promoting birth preparedness involves helping families plan for safe deliveries. This includes identifying a skilled birth attendant, arranging transportation to a healthcare facility, and having funds set aside for any unexpected medical expenses. Additionally, educating families about potential complications and the actions to take in case of emergencies is crucial.
- *Quality Improvement Initiatives:* Implementing quality improvement initiatives within healthcare facilities enhances the overall childbirth experience. This involves addressing issues such as infection control, respectful maternity care, and improved communication between healthcare providers and expectant mothers.
- *Postnatal Care and Newborn Health:* Postnatal care for both mothers and newborns is often overlooked but is vital for ensuring a healthy start. Providing postnatal check-ups, breastfeeding support, and guidance on newborn care helps prevent complications and ensures optimal health for both mother and baby.

Conclusion: Enhancing maternal care and promoting safe childbirth practices are pivotal in building resilient communities in developing nations. Societies can significantly reduce maternal and infant mortality rates by prioritizing skilled birth attendance, antenatal care, emergency obstetric care, maternal health education, community involvement, birth preparedness, and postnatal care. The collaborative effort to ensure safe childbirth practices and comprehensive maternal care sets the foundation for healthier mothers, thriving infants, and, ultimately, more resilient communities.

Childhood Immunization and Nutrition Programs

Childhood immunization and nutrition programs are critical for preventing infectious diseases and supporting optimal growth and development in children. Vaccines protect children from life-threatening diseases such as measles, polio, and pneumonia. Ensuring high immunization coverage through routine vaccination and outreach campaigns is essential in reducing childhood morbidity and mortality [3, 4].

Nutrition plays a crucial role in early childhood development. Exclusive breastfeeding during the first six months provides essential nutrients and protects against infections. Complementary feeding and micronutrient supplementation support healthy growth and cognitive development in children. Effective community-based health education and engagement are vital for increasing awareness about the importance of immunization and nutrition. Empowering caregivers with knowledge and understanding of proper feeding practices can foster healthier habits in children's early years [3, 4]. This section explores the multifaceted strategies that can be employed to enhance maternal care and foster safe childbirth practices, ultimately contributing to healthier mothers and thriving infants.

- *Antenatal Care:* Early and regular antenatal care is crucial for monitoring the health of both the mother and the developing fetus. Community health workers can play a pivotal role in providing antenatal education, promoting healthy behaviors, and identifying potential complications that require medical intervention.
- *Skilled Birth Attendance:* Encouraging skilled birth attendance by trained healthcare professionals, such as midwives or doctors, significantly reduces the risks associated with childbirth. Providing access to trained birth attendants ensures that deliveries take place in a safe and sterile environment, reducing maternal and neonatal mortality rates.
- *Health Facility Upgradation:* Investing in the infrastructure and capacity of health facilities, particularly in rural and underserved areas, is crucial for safe deliveries. Equipping these facilities with necessary medical supplies, personnel, and emergency obstetric care can enhance the likelihood of positive maternal and neonatal outcomes.
- *Emergency Obstetrics Care:* Ensuring access to emergency obstetric care is essential for handling complications during childbirth. Establishing referral networks and transport systems that can swiftly transfer women in need of specialized care to higher-level healthcare facilities can save lives.
- *Promotion of Birth Preparedness:* Educating expectant mothers and their families about the importance of birth preparedness helps them anticipate

potential challenges and make informed decisions. This includes identifying a skilled birth attendant, planning transportation to a health facility, and saving funds for any unexpected medical expenses.

- *Community-Based Interventions:* Empowering communities with knowledge about maternal health and safe childbirth practices can lead to improved health-seeking behaviors. Community health workers can conduct workshops, health camps, and awareness campaigns to disseminate information and foster a supportive environment.
- *Maternal Nutrition:* Promoting proper maternal nutrition during pregnancy is essential for both the mother's health and the development of the fetus. Providing education on balanced diets, micronutrient supplementation, and avoiding harmful practices contributes to healthier pregnancies and better birth outcomes.
- *Postnatal Care:* Postnatal care is often overlooked but is critical for monitoring the health of both the mother and the newborn in the crucial weeks after childbirth. Offering postnatal visits, breastfeeding support, and guidance on newborn care can prevent complications and ensure a healthy start for infants.

Conclusion: Enhancing maternal care and promoting safe childbirth practices are pivotal in building resilient communities within developing nations. Societies can significantly reduce maternal and infant mortality rates by prioritizing early and regular antenatal care, skilled birth attendance, health facility upgradation, emergency obstetric care, and community education. The concerted effort to create an environment where mothers receive appropriate care during pregnancy, childbirth, and the postnatal period ensures that both mothers and infants thrive, setting the foundation for healthier and more resilient communities.

Preventing and Managing Common Childhood Illnesses

Childhood illnesses pose significant challenges to the well-being of communities in developing nations. Effective prevention and management of these illnesses are crucial for building resilient communities. Preventing and managing common childhood illnesses is essential for reducing child mortality and promoting well-being. Acute respiratory infections, diarrhea, and malaria are among the leading causes of childhood morbidity and mortality in developing nations. Community-based integrated management of childhood illnesses (IMCI) programs equip healthcare workers and caregivers with the skills to promptly identify and treat common childhood illnesses. IMCI focuses on early recognition of danger signs, appropriate treatment, and timely referrals to higher-level healthcare facilities when necessary [5, 6].

Preventive measures, such as proper hygiene practices and sanitation, can reduce the incidence of childhood illnesses. Access to safe drinking water and improved sanitation facilities also play a crucial role in preventing waterborne diseases. This section delves into the strategies that can be employed to prevent and manage common childhood illnesses, thus contributing to healthier and more vibrant societies [5, 6].

- *Immunization Programs:* Immunization remains a cornerstone in preventing common childhood illnesses. Comprehensive vaccination schedules protect children against diseases such as measles, polio, diphtheria, and pertussis. Community-wide awareness campaigns, supported by skilled healthcare workers, ensure optimal vaccine coverage.
- *Exclusive Breastfeeding:* Promoting exclusive breastfeeding during the first six months of life provides infants with essential nutrients and antibodies that protect against infections. Community health workers can educate mothers on the benefits of breastfeeding and offer support to overcome challenges.
- *Nutrition Education:* Educating caregivers about proper infant and child nutrition helps prevent malnutrition and related illnesses. Community workshops can teach families about balanced diets, appropriate complementary feeding, and micronutrient-rich foods.
- *Hygiene and Sanitation Practices:* Improving hygiene and sanitation practices within communities reduces the risk of infectious diseases. Education on handwashing, safe food preparation, and proper waste disposal can prevent illnesses caused by contaminated water and food.
- *Integrated Case Management:* Training healthcare providers and community health workers in integrated case management equips them to diagnose and treat common childhood illnesses promptly. This includes conditions like diarrhea, pneumonia, and malaria, which are major causes of childhood morbidity and mortality.
- *Oral Rehydration Therapy:* Promoting the use of oral rehydration solution (ORS) for managing diarrhea prevents dehydration and related complications. Educating caregivers about ORS usage and zinc supplementation supports effective home-based treatment.
- *Early Recognition of Danger Signs:* Empowering parents and caregivers to recognize danger signs in sick children is vital. Educational campaigns can teach them to identify symptoms requiring urgent medical attention, such as difficulty breathing or persistent high fever.
- *Community Health Workers:* Community health workers play a pivotal role in preventing and managing childhood illnesses. These trained individuals can conduct home visits, provide health education, administer basic treatments, and refer severe cases to healthcare facilities.

- *Local Herbal Practices and Traditional Knowledge:* Incorporating local herbal practices and traditional knowledge into healthcare programs respects cultural beliefs while ensuring that safe and effective remedies are used. Collaboration between traditional healers and healthcare providers can help bridge the gap between modern and traditional medicine.

In conclusion, preventing and managing common childhood illnesses is integral to building resilient communities in developing nations. By prioritizing immunization, exclusive breastfeeding, hygiene education, integrated case management, and community engagement, societies can significantly reduce childhood morbidity and mortality rates. The concerted effort to create an environment that fosters child health, coupled with targeted interventions and community involvement, contributes to healthier children and more resilient communities overall.

Case Study 11: *Enhancing Maternal Care and Safe Childbirth Practices in Rural Country X.* It looks at the Safe Motherhood Program - A Journey Towards Safer Births.

Introduction: Maternal mortality and inadequate access to quality maternal care remain pressing challenges in rural areas of Country X. To address these issues and improve maternal health outcomes, a Safe Motherhood Program was initiated in a remote village in the country.

Implementation: The Safe Motherhood Program included a comprehensive set of interventions aimed at enhancing maternal care and promoting safe childbirth practices:

1. Skilled Birth Attendants: The program trained and deployed skilled birth attendants to provide antenatal care, support during childbirth, and postnatal care to pregnant women in the village.

2. Community Awareness: Health education sessions were conducted regularly to raise awareness about the importance of prenatal care, safe delivery practices, and recognizing danger signs during pregnancy and childbirth.

3. Birth Preparedness Plans: Pregnant women and their families were encouraged to create birth preparedness plans, outlining the transportation arrangements and identifying nearby healthcare facilities for emergency situations.

4. Birth Centers: A birthing center was established in the village to provide a safe and clean environment for deliveries, reducing the need for women to travel long distances to access healthcare facilities.

Results: The Safe Motherhood Program led to notable improvements in maternal health outcomes in the village. The presence of skilled birth attendants and birthing centers increased the proportion of women delivering with skilled assistance. As a result, maternal mortality rates declined, and the community witnessed healthier mothers and newborns.

Case Study 12: *Childhood Immunization and Nutrition Programs in a Sub-Saharan African Community.* It looks at a 'Comprehensive Child Health Program - Improving Immunization and Nutrition.'

Introduction: Childhood immunization and proper nutrition play pivotal roles in preventing childhood illnesses and ensuring optimal growth and development. In a sub-Saharan African community, a comprehensive child health program was implemented to enhance immunization coverage and address malnutrition among children.

Childhood Immunization and Nutrition Programs:

Implementation: The child health program consisted of a range of interventions to improve immunization rates and nutrition among children:

1. Immunization Outreach: The program organized regular immunization outreach sessions, where healthcare workers traveled to remote areas to administer vaccines to children who might otherwise have limited access to healthcare facilities.

2. Nutrition Support: Community health workers conducted nutrition assessments and provided counseling to mothers on breastfeeding practices, complementary feeding, and preparing nutritious meals for young children.

3. Growth Monitoring: Regular growth monitoring sessions were held to track the growth and development of children. This enabled early detection of malnutrition and timely intervention.

4. Community Engagement: The program engaged community leaders and volunteers to advocate for immunization and nutrition practices. Local cultural practices and beliefs were taken into account to ensure culturally appropriate interventions.

Results: The child health program yielded significant positive outcomes. Immunization coverage rates increased, leading to a decline in vaccine-preventable diseases among children. The nutrition support and growth monitoring sessions contributed to improved nutritional status among young children, reducing the prevalence of malnutrition.

Conclusion: These case studies demonstrate the importance of enhancing maternal care and safe childbirth practices, implementing childhood immunization and nutrition programs, and preventing and managing common childhood illnesses. By addressing these critical aspects of maternal and child health, communities can achieve significant improvements in maternal and child health outcomes. Culturally sensitive interventions, community engagement, and a comprehensive approach are essential for building resilient maternal and child health programs in developing nations.

CONCLUSION

Maternal and child health interventions play a crucial role in building resilient communities in developing nations. By prioritizing maternal care, safe childbirth practices, childhood immunization, nutrition programs, and prevention and management of childhood illnesses, communities can reduce maternal and infant mortality rates, improve health outcomes, and foster healthier and more vibrant societies. Empowering women, engaging communities, and strengthening healthcare systems are essential for achieving sustained progress in maternal and child health and building resilience for future generations.

REFERENCES

[1]   World Health Organization. WHO recommendations on antenatal care for a positive pregnancy experience. World Health Organization, 2016. Available from: https://apps.who.int/iris/bitstream/handle/10665/250796/9789241549912-eng.pdf

[2]   Kassebaum NJ, Barber RM, Bhutta ZA, *et al.* Global, regional, and national levels of maternal mortality, 1990–2015: a systematic analysis for the Global Burden of Disease Study 2015. Lancet 2016; 388(10053): 1775-812.
[http://dx.doi.org/10.1016/S0140-6736(16)31470-2] [PMID: 27733286]

[3]   World Health Organization. Immunization Coverage. World Health Organization, 2023. Available from: https://www.who.int/news-room/fact-sheets/detail/immunization-coverage

[4]   Victora CG, Bahl R, Barros AJD, *et al.* Breastfeeding in the 21st century: epidemiology, mechanisms, and lifelong effect. Lancet 2016; 387(10017): 475-90.
[http://dx.doi.org/10.1016/S0140-6736(15)01024-7] [PMID: 26869575]

[5]   World Health Organization. Handbook: IMCI integrated management of childhood illness. World Health Organization, 2005. Available from: https://apps.who.int/iris/handle/10665/42939

[6]   Liu L, Oza S, Hogan D, *et al.* Global, regional, and national causes of under-5 mortality in 2000–15: an updated systematic analysis with implications for the Sustainable Development Goals. Lancet 2016; 388(10063): 3027-35.
[http://dx.doi.org/10.1016/S0140-6736(16)31593-8] [PMID: 27839855]

CHAPTER 8

Healthcare Infrastructure and Access

Abstract: Access to quality healthcare is a fundamental human right and a critical determinant of overall well-being, yet many developing nations face significant challenges in healthcare infrastructure and access. This chapter explores strategies to strengthen healthcare facilities and systems, address barriers to healthcare access, and leverage telemedicine and innovative healthcare delivery models to improve access and equity. By prioritizing these interventions, communities can achieve universal healthcare coverage, improve health outcomes, and build resilience.

Keywords: Community health, Health equity, Healthcare access, Healthcare infrastructure, Innovative healthcare delivery models, Telemedicine.

INTRODUCTION

A robust healthcare infrastructure is essential for providing accessible and effective healthcare services. This section emphasizes upgrading and expanding healthcare facilities, training and retaining healthcare workers, implementing health information systems, strengthening primary healthcare, and enhancing emergency preparedness. By prioritizing these strategies, communities can improve health outcomes and resilience, laying the foundation for equitable healthcare access.

Various barriers hinder individuals and communities from accessing healthcare services, exacerbating public health challenges. This section explores strategies to overcome financial, geographical, cultural, and social barriers, including implementing health insurance schemes, mobile health clinics, culturally competent care, and supply chain improvements. By addressing these challenges, societies can ensure equitable access to healthcare services and promote community well-being.

Telemedicine and innovative healthcare delivery models offer promising solutions to expand healthcare access, especially in resource-limited settings. This section highlights the benefits of telemedicine, mobile health initiatives, community health worker networks, e-pharmacies, health kiosks, artificial intelligence in diagnostics, and public-private partnerships. By embracing technology and innovative approaches, communities can transcend barriers to healthcare access and build resilient healthcare systems capable of addressing complex public health challenges.

Strengthening Healthcare Facilities and Systems

A robust healthcare infrastructure is essential for providing accessible and effective healthcare services to communities. Strengthening healthcare facilities and systems is pivotal for creating resilient communities in developing nations; it involves several key strategies. Access to quality healthcare services forms the foundation for addressing public health challenges. This section delves into the multifaceted strategies that can be employed to enhance healthcare infrastructure and systems, contributing to improved health outcomes and community resilience [1, 2].

- *Upgrading and Expanding Healthcare Facilities:* Investments in upgrading and expanding healthcare facilities, especially in underserved regions, are crucial to meet the increasing demand for healthcare services. This includes constructing new health centers, upgrading existing hospitals, and ensuring adequate medical equipment and supplies.
- *Training and Retaining Healthcare Workforce:* The availability of skilled healthcare professionals is vital to providing quality care. Training programs for healthcare workers, including doctors, nurses, and community health workers, can enhance their competencies. Additionally, efforts to retain healthcare personnel in rural and remote areas through incentives and career development opportunities are essential to address workforce shortages.
- *Implementing Health Information Systems:* Effective health information systems facilitate data collection, analysis, and decision-making. Implementing electronic health records and integrating health data across facilities can improve patient care coordination and enable better healthcare planning and resource allocation.
- *Strengthening Primary Healthcare:* A strong primary healthcare system acts as the foundation for a well-functioning healthcare system. It focuses on preventive services, health promotion, and early detection of diseases. By providing comprehensive and integrated care, primary healthcare can reduce the burden on secondary and tertiary facilities.
- *Infrastructure Development:* Investment in healthcare infrastructure is essential for providing comprehensive and effective care. Upgrading existing facilities and building new healthcare centers in underserved areas ensures that communities have physical access to healthcare services, including preventive, curative, and rehabilitative care.

- *Equipping Health Facilities:* Equipping healthcare facilities with essential medical equipment, supplies, and medications is crucial for delivering quality care. Adequate resources enable healthcare providers to offer timely and accurate diagnoses, treatment, and interventions.
- *Human Resources Development:* A well-trained and motivated healthcare workforce is a cornerstone of strong healthcare systems. Developing training programs for healthcare professionals, including doctors, nurses, midwives, and community health workers, improves their capacity to address a wide range of health needs.
- *Task Shifting and Delegation:* Maximizing the skills of healthcare workers through task shifting and delegation can enhance the efficiency of healthcare delivery. Training non-specialized workers to perform certain tasks under appropriate supervision can optimize the use of available human resources.
- *Integrated Health Information Systems:* Implementing integrated health information systems streamlines patient care and management. Electronic health records, telemedicine platforms, and data analytics improve coordination among healthcare providers, facilitate patient tracking, and enable evidence-based decision-making.
- *Community-Based Healthcare Models:* Integrating community-based healthcare models empowers local communities to take ownership of their health. Community health workers play a vital role in delivering basic healthcare services, promoting health education, and facilitating referrals to higher-level facilities.
- *Emergency Preparedness and Response:* Strengthening healthcare systems includes enhancing emergency preparedness and response capabilities. Training healthcare workers to handle emergencies, stockpiling emergency supplies, and developing protocols for disaster response ensure timely interventions during crises.
- *Public-Private Partnerships:* Collaborations between the public and private sectors can improve healthcare access and service quality. Public-private partnerships involve utilizing private healthcare facilities to alleviate the burden on public hospitals and clinics, thereby expanding healthcare access.
- *Health Financing and Insurance:* Implementing effective health financing mechanisms, such as community-based health insurance or government-sponsored insurance programs, helps ensure that healthcare services are financially accessible to all members of the community.
- *Quality Assurance and Accreditation:* Establishing quality assurance mechanisms and accreditation standards ensures that healthcare facilities adhere to defined guidelines and provide safe, effective, and patient-centered care.

Conclusion: Strengthening healthcare facilities and systems is fundamental for building resilient communities in developing nations. By prioritizing infrastructure development, healthcare workforce training, integrated information systems, community engagement, and emergency preparedness, societies can ensure equitable access to quality healthcare services. The collaborative effort to enhance healthcare delivery systems sets the stage for healthier populations, improved health outcomes, and, ultimately, more resilient communities capable of navigating complex public health challenges [1, 2].

Addressing Barriers to Healthcare Access

Ensuring equitable access to healthcare services is critical to building resilient communities in developing nations. Various barriers hinder individuals and communities from accessing healthcare, exacerbating public health challenges. Several barriers hinder access to healthcare services in developing nations. This section explores the multifaceted strategies that can be employed to address barriers to healthcare access, promoting health equity and community well-being. Addressing these challenges is essential to improve healthcare access and equity [3, 4]:

- *Financial Barriers:* High out-of-pocket expenses can be a significant barrier to healthcare access, especially for low-income individuals. Implementing health insurance schemes and social protection programs can help reduce financial barriers and ensure that healthcare services are affordable for all.
- *Geographical Barriers:* In rural and remote areas, geographical distance can pose challenges in accessing healthcare facilities. Mobile health clinics, community health worker programs, and telemedicine initiatives can help bridge the gap and bring essential healthcare services closer to communities.
- *Cultural and Social Barriers:* Cultural beliefs and practices may influence healthcare-seeking behaviors. Culturally competent healthcare services, delivered with sensitivity to local customs and beliefs, can enhance the acceptance and utilization of healthcare services.
- *Gender Disparities:* Gender disparities can affect access to healthcare, particularly for women and girls. Promoting gender equality and empowering women in healthcare decision-making can help address these disparities.
- *Health Literacy:* Limited health literacy can hinder individuals' understanding of health information and treatment plans. Public health campaigns using simple language, visual aids, and community health workers as educators can enhance health literacy and empower individuals to make informed decisions.
- *Social Stigma and Discrimination:* Stigma surrounding certain health conditions, such as HIV/AIDS or mental health disorders, can discourage people from seeking care. Community awareness campaigns, anti-stigma initiatives, and counseling services contribute to reducing stigma and promoting open dialogue.

- *Lack of Awareness:* Many individuals are unaware of available healthcare services and their entitlements. Implementing information campaigns through radio, community meetings, and local media can educate communities about available healthcare options.
- *Supply Chain and Medication Availability:* Inadequate supply chains can lead to shortages of medications and medical supplies. Strengthening supply chains, improving procurement processes, and collaborating with pharmaceutical companies can ensure a consistent and reliable stock of essential medicines.
- *Infrastructure and Transportation:* Lack of transportation infrastructure can hinder people from reaching healthcare facilities. Developing road networks, providing community transportation options, and locating healthcare facilities strategically can enhance accessibility.
- *Health Facility Quality and Acceptability:* Perceptions of poor-quality healthcare services and disrespectful treatment can deter people from seeking care. Ensuring healthcare facilities offer quality services, respectful care, and patient-centered approaches can build trust and increase healthcare utilization.

Conclusion: Addressing barriers to healthcare access is a fundamental step toward building resilient communities in developing nations. By prioritizing strategies that address geographical, financial, cultural, and social barriers, societies can ensure equitable access to healthcare services. The collaborative effort to break down these barriers fosters healthier populations, improved health outcomes, and, ultimately, more resilient communities capable of navigating complex public health challenges [3, 4].

Telemedicine and Innovative Healthcare Delivery Models

Telemedicine and innovative healthcare delivery models offer promising solutions to expand healthcare access, especially in resource-limited settings. In the quest to build resilient communities in developing nations, leveraging technology and innovative healthcare delivery models is crucial for overcoming barriers to healthcare access. This section explores how telemedicine and novel healthcare delivery approaches can transform healthcare delivery, promote equitable access, and enhance community well-being [5, 6]:

- *Telemedicine/Teleconsultations:* Telemedicine revolutionizes healthcare delivery and involves using technology to deliver healthcare services remotely. Through teleconsultations, patients can interact with healthcare providers in real time, receive medical advice, and discuss treatment options without needing physical visits. This approach bridges geographical gaps, especially in remote or underserved areas with scarce healthcare facilities.

○ *Real-Time Consultations:* Telemedicine enables patients to consult with healthcare professionals *via* video calls, allowing for accurate diagnosis, prescription, and follow-up care.

○ *Remote Monitoring:* Telemedicine platforms can track patients' vital signs, chronic conditions, and post-operative recovery, enabling healthcare providers to intervene promptly when necessary.

○ *Medical Education and Training:* Telemedicine can be used to train and update healthcare workers in distant areas, ensuring they remain up to date with the latest medical advancements.

- *Mobile Health (mHealth) Initiatives:* mHealth initiatives leverage mobile technology to deliver healthcare information and services. Text messages, smartphone applications, and telemonitoring devices enable health promotion, disease management, and appointment reminders, improving healthcare access and adherence to treatment.

- *Community Health Worker Networks:* Empowering community health workers with smartphones or tablets equipped with medical apps enhances their capabilities. They can collect and transmit health data, conduct remote consultations, and provide health education to communities.

- *E-Pharmacies and Medication Delivery:* E-pharmacies enable patients to order medications online and have them delivered to their doorstep. This approach addresses medication shortages, improves adherence, and reduces the need for in-person visits.

- *Health Kiosks and Teleclinics:* Setting up health kiosks or teleclinics in rural or urban areas lacking healthcare facilities provides a space for remote consultations and diagnostic tests, connecting patients with specialized doctors.

- *Artificial Intelligence (AI) and Diagnostics:* AI-powered diagnostic tools can analyze medical images and data, assisting healthcare providers in making accurate diagnoses, especially when specialized expertise is limited.

- *Public-Private Partnerships for Technology Adoption:* Collaborations between public health agencies and private technology companies can drive the adoption of telemedicine and innovative solutions. This can include training healthcare workers, providing infrastructure, and offering technical support.

- *Regulatory Framework and Data Security:* Establishing a regulatory framework for telemedicine ensures quality and patient safety. Additionally, safeguarding patient data privacy and security is crucial in maintaining trust in these platforms.

Conclusion: Telemedicine and innovative healthcare delivery models hold the potential to revolutionize healthcare access in developing nations. By embracing technology, fostering partnerships, and addressing regulatory challenges, societies can transcend geographical, financial, and infrastructural barriers. The integration of these approaches empowers communities, enhances healthcare delivery, and contributes to building resilient communities that effectively navigate public health challenges [5, 6].

Case Study 13: *Strengthening Healthcare Facilities and Systems in Rural Country X.* This examines 'The Country X's Health System Strengthening Initiative.'

Introduction: In many rural areas of Country X, limited healthcare facilities and resources have posed significant challenges in providing essential healthcare services to the population. To address these gaps and enhance healthcare infrastructure and access, Country X launched a comprehensive Health System Strengthening Initiative.

Implementation: The Health System Strengthening Initiative involved several key strategies to improve healthcare facilities and systems in rural areas:

1. Infrastructure Development: The initiative focused on constructing and renovating healthcare facilities, including health centers and district hospitals, to ensure they were adequately equipped to deliver quality healthcare services.

2. Human Resource Capacity Building: Training and capacity-building programs were conducted for healthcare professionals to enhance their skills and competencies in providing comprehensive healthcare services.

3. Supply Chain Management: Improved supply chain systems were implemented to ensure the consistent availability of essential medicines, medical equipment, and supplies at healthcare facilities.

4. Information Systems: Health information systems were strengthened to support data collection, analysis, and decision-making, enabling evidence-based planning and resource allocation.

Results: The Health System Strengthening Initiative resulted in significant improvements in healthcare infrastructure and access in rural Country X. The increased number of functional health centers and hospitals, along with enhanced human resource capacity, contributed to improved healthcare service delivery and better health outcomes for the population.

Case Study 14: *Addressing Barriers to Healthcare Access in a Remote Indigenous Community.* This examines 'The Indigenous Health Outreach Program - Breaking Barriers, Providing Care.'

Introduction: Indigenous communities in remote regions often face substantial barriers to accessing healthcare services due to geographical isolation, cultural differences, and inadequate resources. To address these barriers and improve healthcare access, an Indigenous Health Outreach Program was initiated in a remote community.

Implementation: The Indigenous Health Outreach Program focused on several strategies to address barriers to healthcare access in the community:

1. Community-Based Clinics: Mobile healthcare teams comprising healthcare professionals and community health workers conducted regular visits to the remote community, setting up temporary clinics to provide healthcare services.

2. Culturally Sensitive Care: The program ensured that healthcare services were delivered with cultural sensitivity, taking into account the community's customs, beliefs, and language.

3. Health Education and Awareness: Community health workers conducted health education sessions to raise awareness about preventive care, maternal and child health, and common health issues prevalent in the community.

4. Transportation Support: The program provided transportation support to individuals who needed to travel to larger healthcare facilities for specialized care or emergencies.

Results: The Indigenous Health Outreach Program led to notable improvements in healthcare access for the remote indigenous community. The provision of culturally sensitive care, along with regular outreach clinics, increased healthcare utilization among community members. The program facilitated early detection and management of health conditions, leading to improved health outcomes in the community.

Conclusion: These case studies illustrate the significance of strengthening healthcare facilities and systems, addressing barriers to healthcare access, and adopting innovative healthcare delivery models. By implementing targeted strategies, such as infrastructure development, human resource capacity building, and community-based outreach programs, healthcare infrastructure and access can be significantly improved in both rural and remote settings. Culturally appropriate and innovative approaches play a pivotal role in breaking down barriers and ensuring equitable access to quality healthcare for all populations in developing nations.

CONCLUSION

Access to quality healthcare is essential for building resilient communities in developing nations. By strengthening healthcare facilities and systems, addressing barriers to access, and leveraging telemedicine and innovative delivery models, societies can achieve universal healthcare coverage, improve health outcomes, and promote health equity. The collaborative effort to enhance healthcare access sets the stage for healthier populations, improved well-being, and more resilient communities capable of navigating future challenges.

REFERENCES

[1]   World Health Organization. Monitoring the Building Blocks of Health Systems: A Handbook of Indicators and their Measurement Strategies. World Health Organization, 2017. Available from: https://apps.who.int/iris/handle/10665/258734?show=full

[2]   Kotagal M, Lee P, Habiyakare C, *et al.* Improving quality in resource poor settings: observational study from rural Rwanda. BMJ 2009; 339(oct30 1): b3488.
        [http://dx.doi.org/10.1136/bmj.b3488] [PMID: 19880528]

[3]   Xu K, Evans DB, Kadama P, *et al.* Understanding the impact of eliminating user fees: Utilization and catastrophic health expenditures in Uganda. Soc Sci Med 2006; 62(4): 866-76.
        [http://dx.doi.org/10.1016/j.socscimed.2005.07.004] [PMID: 16139936]

[4]   Briggs CJ, Capdegelle P, Garner P. Strategies for integrating primary health services in middle- and low-income countries: effects on performance, costs and patient outcomes. Cochrane Database Syst Rev 2001; (4): CD003318.
        [http://dx.doi.org/10.1002/14651858.CD003318] [PMID: 11687187]

[5]   World Health Organization. (2010). Telemedicine: Opportunities and Developments in Member States. World Health Organization, 2010. Available from: https://www.afro.who.int/publications/telemedicine-opportunities-and-developments-member-state

[6]   World Health Organization. mHealth: New Horizons for Health Through Mobile Technologies. World Health Organization, 2011. Available from: https://www.afro.who.int/publications/mhealth-ne--horizons-health-through-mobile-technologie

CHAPTER 9

Water, Sanitation, and Hygiene (WASH) Interventions

Abstract: Access to clean water, adequate sanitation, and proper hygiene practices are crucial for safeguarding public health and promoting community well-being, especially in developing nations. This chapter emphasizes the importance of WASH interventions in preventing diseases, improving health outcomes, and enhancing resilience within communities. By implementing comprehensive WASH programs and addressing barriers to access, societies can achieve significant progress toward ensuring universal access to clean water and sanitation, thereby creating healthier and more equitable environments for all.

Keywords: Community well-being, Disease prevention, Hygiene, Public health, Sanitation, Water, WASH interventions.

INTRODUCTION

Clean water and sanitation are fundamental human rights essential for preventing waterborne diseases, promoting child health and development, and enhancing overall community well-being. This section highlights the multifaceted significance of WASH interventions in bolstering public health, addressing gender disparities, reducing diarrheal diseases, improving nutrition, and boosting economic productivity. By prioritizing access to clean water and sanitation facilities, societies can create healthier and more equitable environments, fostering sustainable development and resilience.

Effective implementation of WASH programs requires a comprehensive approach that involves infrastructure development, behavior change communication, capacity building, and community engagement. This section explores strategies for successful WASH program implementation, including infrastructure development, behavior change communication, capacity building, and integration with health and education services. By adopting a holistic approach and involving local communities, societies can achieve sustainable improvements in access to clean water, sanitation, and hygiene, thereby promoting public health and community well-being.

WASH interventions have significant effects on disease prevention, child health, economic productivity, and community dignity. This section examines the far-reaching impacts of WASH interventions on disease prevention, maternal and child health, school attendance, economic productivity, and community well-being. By prioritizing WASH interventions and aligning them with the Sustainable Development Goals, societies can create healthier, more resilient communities capable of addressing public health challenges and achieving sustainable development.

Importance of Clean Water and Sanitation for Public Health

Clean water and sanitation are fundamental human rights that underpin various aspects of public health. Access to clean water, sanitation, and hygiene (WASH) services is a fundamental cornerstone of resilient communities in developing nations. The provision of safe water, proper sanitation facilities, and hygiene practices is central to preventing the spread of diseases, promoting overall health, and enhancing community well-being. This section delves into the multifaceted significance of WASH interventions in bolstering public health and community resilience [1, 2].

- *Preventing Waterborne Diseases:* Access to safe drinking water is vital in preventing waterborne diseases such as cholera, typhoid, and diarrheal illnesses. Contaminated water sources can harbor pathogens that lead to severe health consequences, particularly for children and vulnerable populations.
- *Sanitation and Hygiene:* Adequate sanitation facilities, including toilets and proper waste disposal systems, are essential for preventing the spread of diseases. Proper hygiene practices, such as handwashing, can significantly reduce the transmission of infectious agents and improve overall health.
- *Impact on Child Health and Development:* Clean water and sanitation directly affect child health and development. Lack of access to clean water and proper sanitation can lead to stunted growth, malnutrition, and increased susceptibility to diseases in children, impairing their physical and cognitive development.
- *Gender and Social Equity:* Women and girls are disproportionately affected by inadequate WASH facilities, as they are often responsible for water collection and sanitation tasks. Improving WASH access can empower women and promote gender equity.
- *Reducing Diarrheal Diseases:* Diarrheal diseases, primarily caused by poor sanitation and contaminated water, contribute significantly to childhood mortality. Adequate sanitation facilities, coupled with proper waste disposal and handwashing practices, prevent the transmission of pathogens that cause diarrhea.

- *Malnutrition:* Safe water and proper sanitation improve food safety and preparation, reducing the risk of foodborne diseases that can lead to malnutrition, especially among vulnerable populations such as children and pregnant women.
- *Minimizing Water-Related Infections:* Water-related infections, including skin and eye infections, can result from inadequate personal hygiene and the use of contaminated water. Proper hygiene practices, such as regular handwashing and bathing, prevent the spread of infections.
- *Improving Maternal and Child Health:* Access to clean water and sanitation facilities is essential for safe childbirth and postnatal care. Proper sanitation reduces the risk of infections during delivery, and clean water improves hygiene practices, benefiting both mothers and newborns.
- *Enhancing School Attendance and Performance:* Providing clean water and sanitation facilities in schools improves attendance rates and creates a conducive environment for learning. Reduced illness and improved hygiene positively impact students' overall well-being and academic performance.
- *Boosting Economic Productivity:* Healthier communities result in increased economic productivity. When individuals spend less time being sick and caring for sick family members, they can allocate more time to work, education, and income-generating activities.
- *Community Well-Being and Dignity:* Access to clean water and sanitation facilities preserves the dignity of individuals and communities. Clean surroundings, proper waste management, and well-maintained sanitation facilities contribute to a higher quality of life.
- *Preparedness for Health Emergencies:* Communities with established WASH infrastructure are better prepared to respond to health emergencies, including disease outbreaks and natural disasters. Adequate sanitation and hygiene practices mitigate the spread of infections during crises.
- *Sustainable Development Goals (SDGs):* WASH interventions align with the United Nations Sustainable Development Goals, specifically Goal 6, which aims to ensure the availability and sustainable management of water and sanitation for all.

Conclusion: The significance of clean water, sanitation, and hygiene for public health cannot be overstated. By prioritizing WASH interventions, societies can prevent diseases, enhance maternal and child health, improve education, and promote overall well-being. Integrating WASH practices contributes to building resilient communities that are better equipped to address public health challenges and create a healthier, more prosperous future.

Implementing WASH Programs in Developing Communities

Implementing effective WASH programs in developing communities requires a comprehensive and multifaceted approach; it is paramount for building resilient communities in developing nations. Access to clean water, proper sanitation facilities, and improved hygiene practices are crucial for promoting public health and preventing the spread of diseases. This section delves into the multifaceted strategies and considerations involved in successfully implementing WASH programs to enhance the well-being of communities [3, 4].

- *Infrastructure Development:* Investments in water supply infrastructure, such as piped water systems, boreholes, and wells, are crucial in providing clean and accessible water to communities. Similarly, improving sanitation facilities, including toilets and latrines, is essential for promoting safe waste disposal.
- *Behavior Change Communication (BCC):* Behavior change communication is a cornerstone of successful WASH programs. Community engagement and education campaigns can raise awareness about the importance of clean water, sanitation, and hygiene practices, motivating behavior change at the individual and community levels.
- *Capacity Building:* Empowering communities and local institutions with the knowledge and skills to manage and maintain WASH infrastructure is critical for sustainability. Training community members and local leaders to operate and repair water systems and sanitation facilities ensures long-term effectiveness.
- *Integration with Health and Education Services:* Integrating WASH interventions with health and education services can amplify their impact. Incorporating hygiene education into school curricula and healthcare settings can foster lifelong hygiene practices and behavior change.
- Community Engagement and Participation: Engaging the community from the outset is vital. Local input helps tailor WASH interventions to the community's unique needs, culture, and preferences. Involving community members in decision-making and implementation fosters ownership and sustainability.
- Assessment and Needs Identification: Conducting thorough assessments of the community's water sources, sanitation facilities, and hygiene practices is essential. This provides a clear understanding of existing challenges, gaps, and opportunities for improvement.
- Multi-Sectoral Collaboration: WASH programs often require collaboration among various sectors, including health, education, environment, and local governance. Coordinating efforts ensures comprehensive and holistic solutions.
- Hygiene Promotion and Education: Educational initiatives raise awareness about the links between hygiene practices and health outcomes. Empowering communities with knowledge about disease transmission and prevention builds a foundation for healthier behaviors.

- Safe Water Supply: Improving access to safe water sources, which may involve constructing wells, boreholes, or water treatment systems, ensures that communities have a reliable supply of clean water for drinking, cooking, and hygiene.
- Sanitation Facilities: Building or upgrading sanitation facilities, such as latrines or toilets, prevents open defecation and improves privacy and dignity. Facilities should be culturally acceptable, accessible, and gender-sensitive.
- Monitoring and Evaluation: Continuous monitoring and evaluation are essential to assess the effectiveness and sustainability of WASH interventions. Regular data collection helps identify challenges and opportunities for improvement.
- Sustainability and Maintenance: Engaging communities in the ongoing maintenance of infrastructure and hygiene practices is crucial. Implementing strategies for long-term funding, community ownership, and regular maintenance ensures program sustainability.
- Scale-Up and Replication: Successfully implemented WASH programs can serve as models for neighboring communities. Sharing lessons learned and best practices facilitates the replication and scaling up of interventions.

Conclusion: Implementing WASH programs in developing communities requires a comprehensive and collaborative approach. By engaging the community, conducting assessments, building capacity, and focusing on behavior change, societies can make significant strides in improving access to clean water, sanitation, and hygiene. The concerted effort to implement sustainable WASH interventions contributes to building resilient communities with better public health outcomes and improved overall well-being.

Impact on Disease Prevention and Community Well-being

WASH interventions have far-reaching effects on disease prevention and community well-being. Water, sanitation, and hygiene (WASH) interventions are integral to building resilient communities in developing nations. These interventions are pivotal in preventing diseases, improving public health outcomes, and enhancing the overall well-being of individuals and communities. This section explores the significant impact of WASH interventions on disease prevention and community well-being [5, 6].

- *Reduction of Waterborne Diseases:* The provision of safe drinking water and improved sanitation facilities can significantly reduce the incidence of waterborne diseases. *WASH interventions that improve water quality and ensure reliable water sources significantly reduce the incidence of waterborne diseases such as cholera, dysentery, and typhoid.* Studies have shown that WASH interventions contribute to substantial declines in diarrheal diseases and related child mortality.

- *Enhanced Nutrition and Growth:* Clean water and sanitation are essential for improving nutrition and promoting healthy growth in children. Adequate access to water supports breastfeeding practices, facilitates food preparation, and ensures food safety.
- *Social and Economic Benefits:* WASH interventions bring about social and economic benefits for communities. Reduced illness and improved productivity result in fewer workdays lost due to sickness, leading to increased economic stability.
- Preventing Diarrhoeal Diseases: Proper sanitation and hygiene practices, including access to improved sanitation facilities and proper waste disposal, are crucial for preventing diarrhoeal diseases. These interventions curb the transmission of pathogens that cause diarrhea, especially in children.
- Curbing Neglected Tropical Diseases: WASH interventions have a direct impact on neglected tropical diseases, such as soil-transmitted helminthiasis and trachoma. By reducing exposure to contaminated soil and promoting personal hygiene, these interventions contribute to disease control.
- Enhancing Maternal and Child Health: Adequate WASH facilities, including clean water and sanitation services, are essential for safe childbirth and postnatal care. Improved maternal health contributes to healthier pregnancies, safer deliveries, and reduced maternal and infant mortality rates.
- Preventing Respiratory Infections: Hygiene practices like proper handwashing and maintaining clean living environments can prevent respiratory infections such as pneumonia and influenza. These practices reduce the transmission of pathogens that cause respiratory illnesses.
- Improving School Attendance and Performance: WASH interventions in schools lead to better attendance rates and improved overall health of students. Children who are not burdened by waterborne diseases or infections can attend school more regularly and concentrate on their studies.
- Enhancing Community Dignity and Well-being: Access to clean water and sanitation facilities preserves the dignity of individuals and communities. A clean and safe environment enhances overall well-being, reduces stigma, and fosters a sense of pride.
- Mitigating Health Emergencies: Communities with improved WASH infrastructure are better equipped to respond to health emergencies. Adequate sanitation and hygiene practices prevent disease outbreaks, especially during crises such as natural disasters or disease epidemics.
- Economic Benefits and Productivity: Healthier communities result in increased economic productivity. Reduced healthcare expenses, increased labor force participation, and improved educational outcomes contribute to economic growth.

- Sustainable Development Goals (SDGs): WASH interventions align with several United Nations Sustainable Development Goals, particularly Goal 3 (Good Health and Well-being) and Goal 6 (Clean Water and Sanitation), contributing to the broader agenda of global development.

Conclusion: The impact of WASH interventions on disease prevention and community well-being cannot be overstated. By prioritizing access to clean water, sanitation facilities, and proper hygiene practices, societies can significantly reduce disease burden, improve public health outcomes, and enhance the overall quality of life for individuals and communities. Integrating WASH practices is a vital step toward building resilient communities capable of navigating public health challenges and achieving sustainable development.

Case Study 15:*Importance of Clean Water and Sanitation for Public Health in a Rural Village in Country X.* It examines 'Clean Water for Healthy Living - The Transformation of a Village in Country X.'

Introduction: Access to clean water and sanitation is a fundamental aspect of public health. In a rural village in Country X, the lack of clean water sources and inadequate sanitation facilities had severe implications for the health and well-being of the community. To address this critical issue and improve public health outcomes, a Clean Water and Sanitation Project was initiated.

Implementation: The Clean Water and Sanitation Project involved several key interventions to provide access to clean water and improve sanitation in the village:

1. Construction of Water Sources: The project established protected water sources, including boreholes and hand pumps, to provide the community with access to clean and safe drinking water.

2. Sanitation Facilities: Improved sanitation facilities, including the construction of latrines and proper waste disposal systems, were implemented to promote hygienic practices.

3. Hygiene Promotion: Community health workers conducted hygiene education sessions to raise awareness about the importance of handwashing, proper sanitation, and safe water handling practices.

4. Community Participation: The community actively participated in the planning and implementation of the project, fostering a sense of ownership and sustainability.

Results: The Clean Water and Sanitation Project led to a transformative impact on public health in the village. Access to clean water and improved sanitation facilities significantly reduced waterborne diseases and gastrointestinal infections. The hygiene education sessions contributed to improved hygienic practices, further preventing the spread of communicable diseases. As a result, the overall health and well-being of the community improved, with fewer cases of water-related illnesses reported.

Case Study 16:*Implementing WASH Programs in a Refugee Settlement in East Africa.* It examines 'Building Health and Hope - WASH Interventions in a Refugee Community.'

Introduction: In refugee settlements, ensuring access to clean water, sanitation, and hygiene facilities is crucial for safeguarding public health, especially in environments with high population density and limited resources. In a refugee settlement in East Africa, a WASH Program was implemented to address the unique challenges faced by the displaced population.

Implementation: The WASH Program in the refugee settlement involved a comprehensive approach to improve water, sanitation, and hygiene conditions:

1. Water Supply: The program focused on establishing water supply systems, including water wells and distribution points, to provide clean and safe water to the settlement residents.

2. Sanitation Facilities: Adequate sanitation facilities, such as communal latrines and bathing areas, were constructed to ensure proper waste disposal and personal hygiene.

3. Hygiene Promotion: Hygiene education campaigns were conducted to raise awareness about proper handwashing techniques, disease prevention, and waste management.

4. Solid Waste Management: The program implemented waste management initiatives to address the environmental impact of waste accumulation and reduce potential health hazards.

Results: The implementation of the WASH Program significantly improved public health conditions in the refugee settlement. Access to clean water and sanitation facilities reduced the prevalence of waterborne diseases, gastrointestinal infections, and other communicable illnesses. Hygiene education fostered behavioral changes, leading to healthier practices within the community. The effective waste management system further contributed to maintaining a clean and hygienic living environment.

Conclusion: These case studies highlight the vital importance of clean water and sanitation for public health and the positive impact of implementing WASH programs in developing communities. By providing access to clean water sources, improving sanitation facilities, and promoting hygiene education, public health conditions can be significantly enhanced, leading to disease prevention and improved community well-being. WASH interventions play a pivotal role in building resilient communities and ensuring healthier living conditions in developing nations, particularly in vulnerable settings such as rural areas and refugee settlements.

CONCLUSION

Access to clean water, adequate sanitation, and proper hygiene practices are essential for promoting public health and community well-being, particularly in developing nations. By implementing comprehensive WASH programs, addressing barriers to access, and prioritizing behavior change communication and community engagement, societies can achieve significant progress toward ensuring universal access to clean water and sanitation. The collective effort to prioritize WASH interventions is crucial for building resilient communities capable of addressing public health challenges and creating healthier and more equitable environments for all.

REFERENCES

[1]   Prüss-Ustün A, Bartram J, Clasen T, *et al.* Burden of disease from inadequate water, sanitation and hygiene in low☐ and middle☐income settings: a retrospective analysis of data from 145 countries. Trop Med Int Health 2014; 19(8): 894-905.
        [http://dx.doi.org/10.1111/tmi.12329] [PMID: 24779548]

[2]   World Health Organization. Drinking-water. World Health Organization, 2022, Available from: https://www.who.int/news-room/fact-sheets/detail/drinking-water

[3]   World Health Organization. WASH in Health Care Facilities: Global Baseline Report 2019. WHO. Available from: https://www.who.int/publications/i/item/9789241515504

[4]   Bartram J, Cairncross S. Hygiene, sanitation, and water: forgotten foundations of health. PLoS Med 2010; 7(11): e1000367.
        [http://dx.doi.org/10.1371/journal.pmed.1000367] [PMID: 21085694]

[5]   Clasen T, Roberts I, Rabie T, Schmidt W, Cairncross S. Interventions to improve water quality for preventing diarrhoea. Cochrane Database Syst Rev 2006; (3): CD004794.
        [http://dx.doi.org/10.1002/14651858.CD004794.pub2] [PMID: 16856059]

[6]   Freeman MC, Greene LE, Dreibelbis R, *et al.* Assessing the impact of a school☐based water treatment, hygiene and sanitation programme on pupil absence in Nyanza Province, Kenya: a cluster☐randomized trial. Trop Med Int Health 2012; 17(3): 380-91.
        [http://dx.doi.org/10.1111/j.1365-3156.2011.02927.x] [PMID: 22175695]

CHAPTER 10

Sustainable Solutions for Nutrition and Food Security

Abstract: Nutrition and food security are essential components of public health and sustainable development, particularly in developing nations. Malnutrition and food insecurity pose significant challenges to individual well-being and community resilience. This chapter explores strategies for addressing these issues, including promoting sustainable agriculture, empowering communities, and strengthening food value chains. By prioritizing nutrition education, women's empowerment, and community engagement, societies can improve health outcomes, foster sustainable development, and create resilient communities capable of overcoming food security challenges.

Keywords: Community empowerment, Food security, Malnutrition, Nutrition, Sustainable agriculture.

INTRODUCTION

Malnutrition and food insecurity are complex challenges with far-reaching health, economic, and social implications. This section outlines strategies for addressing these issues, including promoting nutrient-dense diets, supporting breastfeeding, empowering communities in agriculture, and implementing community-based interventions. By prioritizing access to nutritious food and empowering communities, societies can improve overall well-being and resilience.

Promoting sustainable agriculture and community food initiatives are crucial for achieving food security and improving nutrition. This section discusses agroecological practices, climate-resilient farming, community food gardens, and value chain strengthening. By supporting environmentally friendly farming practices and empowering communities to produce their food, societies can create resilient food systems that ensure access to nutritious food for all.

Empowering communities to take charge of their nutrition is essential for building resilient societies. This section explores strategies for nutrition education, women's empowerment, community-led interventions, and participatory approaches. By involving communities in decision-making and providing practical tools, societies can create lasting changes in dietary habits and promote overall well-being.

Addressing Malnutrition and Food Insecurity

Malnutrition and food insecurity are multifaceted and complex challenges that significantly impact the health and resilience of communities in developing nations. Addressing these issues requires a multifaceted approach that encompasses access to nutritious food, proper feeding practices, health education, and community engagement. This section delves into the strategies and considerations for effectively addressing malnutrition and food insecurity, contributing to improved community well-being [1 - 3].

- Understanding Malnutrition and Food Insecurity: Malnutrition encompasses both undernutrition and overnutrition, including underweight, stunting, wasting, and obesity. Food insecurity refers to limited access to safe and nutritious food. Both issues have far-reaching health, economic, and social implications.
- Promoting Nutrient-Dense Diets: Educating communities about the importance of consuming a variety of nutrient-dense foods is crucial. Encouraging the consumption of fruits, vegetables, whole grains, lean proteins, and dairy products enhances overall nutrition.
- Exclusive Breastfeeding and Complementary Feeding: Promoting exclusive breastfeeding during the first six months of life and introducing nutritious complementary foods thereafter is vital for optimal infant and child growth. This approach provides essential nutrients and antibodies.
- Micronutrient Supplementation: Providing vitamin and mineral supplements, especially to vulnerable populations like pregnant women and children, addresses micronutrient deficiencies that can lead to health complications.
- Agricultural Diversification: Encouraging communities to cultivate a diverse range of crops promotes dietary variety and resilience against food shortages. It also ensures access to a range of essential nutrients.
- Local Food Production and Community Gardens: Establishing community gardens and promoting local food production empowers communities to grow their nutritious foods. This enhances food availability, especially in resource-limited areas.
- School Feeding Programs: Implementing school feeding programs not only improves students' nutrition but also incentivizes school attendance. These programs ensure that children receive at least one nutritious meal per day.
- Income Generation and Livelihood Support: Economic empowerment through income generation and livelihood support initiatives improves families' purchasing power, enabling them to access nutritious foods.

- Nutrition Education: Conducting nutrition education sessions empowers individuals and caregivers to make informed dietary choices. These sessions can cover topics such as balanced diets, portion control, and hygiene practices.
- Community-Based Nutrition Interventions: Engaging community health workers to provide nutrition education, conduct growth monitoring, and offer counselling to support families in improving their nutritional status.
- Partnerships and Collaboration: Collaboration between government agencies, NGOs, community organizations, and the private sector is essential to pool resources, knowledge, and expertise for effective interventions.
- Monitoring and Evaluation: Regularly assessing the impact of interventions through data collection and analysis helps identify successful strategies and areas for improvement.
- *Undernutrition and Micronutrient Deficiencies:* Undernutrition, including stunting, wasting, and micronutrient deficiencies, affects millions of children and adults in developing nations. Lack of access to diverse and nutritious food contributes to impaired growth, weakened immune systems, and developmental delays.
- *Overnutrition and Non-Communicable Diseases:* Besides undernutrition, the rising prevalence of overnutrition, characterized by obesity and diet-related non-communicable diseases (NCDs), poses a significant public health concern. Access to unhealthy and processed foods, coupled with changing dietary patterns, increases the risk of NCDs, such as diabetes and cardiovascular diseases.
- *Food Insecurity and Vulnerable Populations:* Food insecurity, resulting from inadequate food availability, accessibility, and utilization, affects vulnerable populations disproportionately. Women, children, the elderly, and marginalized communities are particularly at risk of food insecurity, leading to adverse health outcomes and reduced productivity.

Conclusion: Addressing malnutrition and food insecurity requires a comprehensive and collaborative approach. By prioritizing nutrient-dense diets, promoting breastfeeding, supporting local food production, and implementing community-based interventions, societies can significantly improve the nutrition and food security of communities. The collective effort to ensure access to nutritious food contributes to building resilient communities that are better equipped to navigate public health challenges and promote the health and well-being of individuals across generations.

Sustainable Agriculture and Community Food Initiatives

Promoting sustainable agriculture and empowering communities with local food initiatives are key components of building resilient communities in developing nations. These approaches ensure a consistent supply of nutritious food, strengthen local economies, and empower individuals to take charge of their well-being. This section delves into the strategies and considerations for fostering sustainable agriculture and community food initiatives to enhance food security and improve nutrition [3, 4].

- *Agroecological Practices:* Agroecological approaches prioritize sustainable and regenerative farming practices that improve soil health, conserve natural resources, and enhance biodiversity. Diverse and resilient agroecosystems provide communities with a steady supply of nutritious food.
- *Climate-Resilient Farming:* Climate change poses challenges to food security, with unpredictable weather patterns affecting agricultural productivity. Encouraging climate-resilient farming techniques, such as drought-resistant crops and water-efficient irrigation, helps mitigate the impact of climate-related disruptions on food production.
- *Community Food Gardens and Urban Agriculture:* Community-based food gardens and urban agriculture initiatives empower communities to grow their food, ensuring greater access to fresh produce. These initiatives promote self-sufficiency, food sovereignty, and community cohesion.
- *Food Value Chain Strengthening:* Enhancing the food value chain, from production to distribution and marketing, improves the availability and affordability of nutritious food. Supporting smallholder farmers, establishing local markets, and reducing food waste contribute to a more inclusive and sustainable food system.
- Sustainable Agriculture Practices: Implementing sustainable farming techniques is crucial for long-term food security and environmental preservation. These practices maximize agricultural output while minimizing negative ecological impacts.
  - *Agroecology: Integrating ecological principles into agriculture helps maintain soil health, conserve water, and reduce the need for chemical inputs. Crop rotation, intercropping, and integrated pest management contribute to a resilient farming ecosystem.*
  - *Conservation Agriculture: Techniques like minimal soil disturbance, permanent soil cover, and diversified crop rotations reduce soil erosion, improve water retention, and enhance crop yields.*
  - *Permaculture: Designing farming systems based on natural ecosystems leads to efficient land use, reduced resource consumption, and increased biodiversity.*
- Seed Banks and Indigenous Crops: Establishing seed banks for indigenous and locally adapted crops preserves biodiversity and enhances resilience against climate change. These crops are often better suited to local conditions and have high nutritional value.

- Crop Diversification: Encouraging farmers to diversify their crops reduces vulnerability to crop failures and improves dietary diversity. It also has economic benefits by offering a variety of produce for the market.
- Agricultural Training and Extension Services: Providing farmers with training in modern and sustainable agricultural techniques equips them with the skills needed to enhance productivity and adapt to changing conditions.
- Women's Empowerment in Agriculture: Empowering women in agriculture contributes to food security. Women often play a significant role in food production and household nutrition, so supporting their access to resources and decision-making is essential.
- Farm-to-Table Initiatives: Promoting direct connections between producers and consumers through farmers' markets, food cooperatives, and farm-to-school programs reduces the distance food travels, ensuring freshness and supporting local economies.
- Value Addition and Food Processing: Encouraging food processing and value addition at the local level extends shelf life, reduces food waste, and creates opportunities for small-scale entrepreneurs.
- Partnerships and Knowledge Sharing: Collaborating with agricultural experts, research institutions, NGOs, and government agencies facilitates the exchange of knowledge and expertise, driving innovation in sustainable agriculture.

Conclusion: Sustainable agriculture and community food initiatives are vital for achieving food security and improving nutrition in developing nations. By promoting environmentally friendly farming practices, empowering communities to grow their food, and fostering collaborations across sectors, societies can build resilient communities that are less reliant on external food sources and better equipped to overcome food security challenges. These initiatives contribute to healthier populations and create a foundation for long-term community well-being.

Empowering Communities to Improve Nutrition

Empowering communities to take charge of their nutrition is a fundamental step toward building resilient communities in developing nations. When individuals are equipped with knowledge, skills, and resources, they can make informed dietary choices, implement healthier practices, and contribute to improved overall well-being. It is essential for sustainable nutrition and food security interventions. This section delves into the strategies and considerations for empowering communities to improve nutrition, leading to healthier populations and enhanced community resilience [5, 6].

- *Nutrition Education and Behavior Change:* Promoting nutrition education at the community level fosters informed food choices and healthy eating habits. Behaviour change campaigns on infant and young child feeding, balanced diets, and food safety empower individuals to make healthier choices for themselves and their families. *Raising awareness about the importance of proper nutrition is the first step toward empowering communities. Nutrition education campaigns should focus on explaining the benefits of balanced diets, essential nutrients, and the impact of various foods on health.*
- *Women's Empowerment:* Empowering women is central to improving nutrition outcomes. Gender-responsive interventions that promote women's access to resources, decision-making power, and nutrition-sensitive programs positively impact maternal and child nutrition.
- *Community-Led Nutrition Interventions:* Community-led nutrition interventions encourage local ownership and participation. Engaging community members in planning and implementing nutrition programs enhances program effectiveness and sustainability.
- *Social Safety Nets and Food Assistance:* Social safety nets and food assistance programs provide critical support to vulnerable populations during times of crisis or food insecurity. Targeted interventions, such as cash transfers or school feeding programs, can alleviate immediate nutritional needs and promote food security.
- Cultural Sensitivity and Local Context: Tailoring nutrition education to the local cultural context enhances relevance and engagement. Understanding traditional food practices and beliefs allows for effective communication of nutritional information.
- Community Workshops and Seminars: Conducting interactive workshops and seminars provides platforms for communities to learn about nutrition, cooking methods, meal planning, and portion control. Hands-on activities foster practical skills.
- Cooking Demonstrations and Recipe Sharing: Organizing cooking demonstrations showcasing nutrient-rich recipes encourages communities to explore new and healthier culinary options. Sharing recipes through community networks promotes sustainable dietary changes.
- Hygiene and Food Safety Training: Education on food safety practices ensures that communities are aware of the risks associated with improper handling and storage of food, reducing the likelihood of foodborne illnesses.
- Local Food Promotion: Highlighting the nutritional value of locally available foods encourages communities to make use of regional resources. This promotes dietary diversity and supports local economies.

- Home Gardening and Nutrition: Encouraging families to cultivate home gardens not only provides access to fresh produce but also educates them about the nutritional benefits of homegrown fruits and vegetables.
- Promoting Breastfeeding and Infant Nutrition: Empowering mothers with knowledge about exclusive breastfeeding, proper complementary feeding, and infant nutrition sets the foundation for optimal growth and development.
- Engaging Community Health Workers: Training and empowering community health workers to provide nutrition counseling and guidance ensures a consistent source of accurate information at the grassroots level.
- Participatory Approaches: Involving community members in planning, designing, and implementing nutrition programs fosters ownership and sustainability. Community-led initiatives are more likely to be embraced and adopted.
- Measuring and Celebrating Progress: Regularly assessing the impact of nutrition interventions, such as growth monitoring in children, creates accountability and motivation for positive behavior change. Celebrating achievements reinforces the value of collective efforts.
- Policy Advocacy and Partnerships: Community advocacy for improved nutrition policies and partnerships with governmental and non-governmental entities amplify the impact of community-led initiatives.

Conclusion: Empowering communities to improve nutrition goes beyond information dissemination; it involves fostering knowledge, skills, and ownership. By involving communities in decision-making, providing practical tools, and promoting culturally relevant practices, societies can create lasting changes in dietary habits and build resilient communities that are proactive in addressing public health challenges. The collective effort toward better nutrition enhances overall community well-being and contributes to a healthier and more prosperous future.

Case Study 17: *Addressing Malnutrition and Food Insecurity in a Sub-Saharan African Village.* It examines 'The Nutrition Revival Program - Nourishing a Village.'

Introduction: Malnutrition and food insecurity are prevalent challenges in many sub-Saharan African communities, affecting the health and well-being of vulnerable populations. In a rural village facing severe food shortages and high rates of malnutrition, the Nutrition Revival Program was initiated to address these pressing issues.

Implementation: The Nutrition Revival Program focused on several strategies to tackle malnutrition and food insecurity in the village:

1. Nutritional Supplementation: The program provided targeted nutritional supplementation to vulnerable groups, such as pregnant women, lactating mothers, and young children, to address immediate nutritional needs.

2. Sustainable Farming Techniques: Training sessions were conducted to educate farmers on sustainable agricultural practices, including crop diversification, soil conservation, and water-efficient farming methods.

3. Community Food Banks: Community food banks were established to store surplus food and distribute it during times of food scarcity, ensuring food availability during lean periods.

4. Kitchen Gardens: The program promoted the establishment of kitchen gardens at household levels, encouraging the cultivation of vegetables and fruits for improved dietary diversity.

Results: The Nutrition Revival Program led to significant improvements in addressing malnutrition and food insecurity in the village. Nutritional supplementation contributed to improved health outcomes among vulnerable groups, reducing the prevalence of malnutrition-related illnesses. The adoption of sustainable farming techniques increased agricultural productivity, leading to greater food availability. Kitchen gardens empowered households to produce nutritious foods locally, promoting dietary diversity and reducing dependency on external food sources. As a result, the overall nutrition status of the community improved, enhancing their resilience to food crises.

Case Study 18: *Sustainable Agriculture and Community Food Initiatives in a Rural Region of Country X.* It looks at 'From Food Scarcity to Food Sovereignty - A Transformational Journey.'

Introduction: In many rural regions of Country X, food scarcity and lack of food sovereignty have been longstanding challenges. In response to these issues, a sustainable agriculture and community food initiatives program was launched to empower communities and improve food security.

Implementation: The sustainable agriculture and community food initiatives program involved several key interventions:

1. Agroecological Farming: The program promoted agroecological farming practices, emphasizing organic farming, agroforestry, and traditional seed preservation methods.

2. Farmer Cooperatives: Farmers were organized into cooperatives to collectively access resources, share knowledge, and market their produce, strengthening their bargaining power.

3. Community Seed Banks: Community seed banks were established to preserve traditional seed varieties, ensuring crop diversity and resilience against climate change.

4. Food Preservation and Processing: Training sessions were conducted on food preservation and processing techniques, enabling communities to store surplus produce and reduce post-harvest losses.

Results: The sustainable agriculture and community food initiatives program led to a transformative journey towards food sovereignty in the rural region. Agroecological farming practices resulted in increased crop yields and enhanced ecological sustainability. The establishment of farmer cooperatives fostered community solidarity and economic empowerment. Community seed banks played a crucial role in preserving indigenous seed varieties, protecting traditional knowledge, and ensuring crop resilience. The acquisition of food preservation and processing skills enabled communities to have access to nutritious foods throughout the year. As a result, the region experienced a significant reduction in food insecurity, with communities attaining greater control over their food production and consumption patterns.

Conclusion: These case studies highlight the importance of addressing malnutrition and food insecurity, promoting sustainable agriculture and community food initiatives, and empowering communities to improve nutrition. By implementing targeted interventions, such as nutritional supplementation, sustainable farming practices, and community-driven food initiatives, public health systems can effectively address malnutrition and food insecurity in developing nations. Empowering communities to take charge of their food production and access fosters greater resilience, improved food security, and enhanced nutrition outcomes, contributing to the overall well-being of populations in vulnerable settings.

CONCLUSION

Addressing malnutrition and food insecurity requires a multifaceted approach that prioritizes access to nutritious food, promotes sustainable agriculture, and empowers communities. By investing in nutrition education, women's empowerment, and community-led initiatives, societies can improve health outcomes, foster sustainable development, and create resilient communities capable of overcoming food security challenges. The collective effort to prioritize nutrition and food security is essential for building a healthier and more prosperous future for all.

REFERENCES

[1]   Black RE, Victora CG, Walker SP, *et al.* Maternal and child undernutrition and overweight in low-income and middle-income countries. Lancet 2013; 382(9890): 427-51.
[http://dx.doi.org/10.1016/S0140-6736(13)60937-X] [PMID: 23746772]

[2]   United Nations. The State of Food Security and Nutrition in the World 2020. Transforming food systems for affordable healthy diets. United Nations, Food and Agriculture Organization (FAO), 2020. Available from: http://www.fao.org/ 3/ca9692en/ca9692en.pdf

[3]   Altieri MA, Nicholls CI. Agroecology Scaling Up for Food Sovereignty and Resiliency. In: Lichtfouse E, Ed. Sustainable Agriculture Reviews Sustainable Agriculture Reviews. Dordrecht: Springer 2012; 11.
[http://dx.doi.org/10.1007/978-94-007-5449-2_1]

[4]   Food and Agriculture Organization of the United Nations (FAO). Climate-Smart Agriculture Sourcebook. Food and Agriculture Organization (FAO), 2013. Available from: http://www. fao.org/3/i3325e/i3325e.pdf

[5]   Bhutta ZA, Das JK, Rizvi A, *et al.* Evidence-based interventions for improvement of maternal and child nutrition: what can be done and at what cost? Lancet 2013; 382(9890): 452-77.
[http://dx.doi.org/10.1016/S0140-6736(13)60996-4] [PMID: 23746776]

[6]   Nisbett N, Gillespie S, Haddad L, Harris J. Why Worry About the Politics of Childhood Undernutrition? World Dev 2014; 64: 420-33.
[http://dx.doi.org/10.1016/j.worlddev.2014.06.018]

CHAPTER 11

Building Resilient Mental Health Support Systems

Abstract: Mental health and psychosocial well-being are crucial aspects of overall health, particularly in developing nations where various socio-economic factors can exacerbate mental health challenges. Recognizing the prevalence and impact of mental health issues, building psychosocial support systems, and integrating mental health into public health programs are essential steps toward promoting resilience and well-being. This chapter explores strategies for recognizing mental health challenges, building effective psychosocial support systems, and integrating mental health into public health programs in developing nations.

Keywords: Developing nations, Mental health, Psychosocial support, Public health, Resilience.

INTRODUCTION

Mental health is an integral part of overall well-being and plays a crucial role in shaping the resilience and productivity of individuals and communities. Mental health challenges in developing nations are influenced by various socio-economic and cultural factors. In developing nations, mental health challenges are prevalent, often exacerbated by poverty, conflict, and limited access to healthcare services. Recognizing the burden of mental disorders, the impact of adversities, and the role of stigma and discrimination is crucial. Addressing mental health challenges requires understanding cultural perceptions, socio-economic factors, and the unique stressors faced by communities. By raising awareness, reducing stigma, and integrating mental health into primary healthcare, societies can promote resilience and well-being.

Psychosocial support systems are essential for promoting mental well-being and resilience in developing nations. Community-based approaches, peer support programs, and culturally sensitive interventions are effective strategies for building psychosocial support systems. By engaging communities, reducing stigma, and integrating psychosocial support into existing services, societies can create inclusive and supportive environments that empower individuals to cope with challenges and thrive.

Integrating mental health into public health programs is vital for addressing the diverse needs of communities in developing nations. Task shifting, policy advocacy, and collaboration between sectors are key strategies for integrating mental health into existing health initiatives. By recognizing the nexus between physical and mental health, strengthening health systems, and promoting early intervention and prevention, societies can build resilient healthcare systems that prioritize mental well-being.

Recognizing Mental Health Challenges in Developing Nations

Mental health challenges are universal, but they manifest uniquely in developing nations due to complex social, economic, and cultural factors. Recognizing these challenges is the first step toward building resilient communities that address mental health issues and promote well-being. This section delves into the importance of recognizing mental health challenges in developing nations and understanding their impact on individuals and communities [1, 2].

- *Burden of Mental Disorders:* Mental disorders, including depression, anxiety, and post-traumatic stress disorder (PTSD), pose a significant burden in developing nations. The lack of adequate resources and stigma associated with mental health issues often leads to underreporting and limited access to care.
- *Impact of Adversities:* Developing nations frequently face challenges such as armed conflicts, natural disasters, and economic instability. These adversities contribute to the development or exacerbation of mental health problems among affected populations.
- *Stigma and Discrimination:* Stigma and discrimination surrounding mental health hinder help-seeking behaviors and access to mental health services. Addressing misconceptions and promoting mental health literacy are essential steps in reducing the stigma associated with mental disorders.
- Cultural Perceptions of Mental Health: In many developing nations, mental health is often stigmatized or misunderstood due to cultural beliefs and misconceptions. Stigma can prevent individuals from seeking help and delay timely interventions.
- Socioeconomic Factors: Poverty, lack of access to education, and limited job opportunities can contribute to stress, anxiety, and depression. Economic instability and inequality exacerbate mental health challenges, creating a vicious cycle.
- Conflict and Displacement: Communities in developing nations frequently face conflict, displacement, and humanitarian crises. These traumatic experiences can lead to post-traumatic stress disorder (PTSD) and other mental health issues.
- Access to Mental Health Services: The shortage of mental health professionals and limited access to quality care are prevalent challenges. Many communities

lack the resources and infrastructure needed to provide comprehensive mental health support.

- Gender-Specific Challenges: Gender-based violence, discrimination, and unequal access to opportunities can contribute to mental health challenges, particularly among women and girls.
- Child and Adolescent Mental Health: Children and adolescents face unique challenges in developing nations, including inadequate access to education, exposure to violence, and limited psychosocial support.
- Stressors Related to Urbanization: Rapid urbanization can lead to social disconnection, increased workload, and lack of support networks, contributing to mental health issues among urban populations.
- Coping with Natural Disasters: Communities in developing nations are often more vulnerable to natural disasters. The aftermath of such events can result in trauma, grief, and increased mental health challenges.
- Strengthening Resilience: Understanding the impact of mental health challenges on community resilience is crucial. When individuals struggle with mental health issues, the community as a whole may face setbacks in economic development and social cohesion.
- Raising Awareness and Reducing Stigma: Promoting awareness campaigns that challenge stigma, increase understanding of mental health, and emphasize the importance of seeking help is essential for initiating positive change.
- Integration with Primary Healthcare: Integrating mental health services into primary healthcare systems helps ensure that individuals can access care as part of their overall health needs.
- Localizing Interventions: Addressing mental health challenges requires interventions that consider cultural norms, local languages, and community-specific approaches to support and care.

Conclusion: Recognising mental health challenges in developing nations is a critical step toward building resilient communities and prioritizing holistic well-being. By understanding the unique socio-cultural factors contributing to these challenges, societies can implement culturally sensitive interventions, reduce stigma, and promote access to mental health services. The collective effort to address mental health challenges contributes to building communities better equipped to navigate public health challenges, support individuals in need, and foster overall community resilience [1, 2].

Building Psychosocial Support Systems

Psychosocial support systems are essential components of resilient communities in developing nations. These systems provide individuals and communities with the tools to cope with adversity, promote mental well-being, and foster a sense of belonging. This section delves into the strategies and considerations for building effective psychosocial support systems that address mental health challenges and strengthen community resilience [3, 4].

- *Community-Based Approaches:* Community-based psychosocial support systems empower individuals and communities to address mental health issues collectively. Utilizing community resources, social networks, and culturally appropriate interventions can strengthen resilience and promote well-being. *Engaging community members in the design, development, and implementation of psychosocial support systems is crucial. Community ownership ensures cultural relevance and acceptance.*
- *Psychosocial First Aid:* Psychosocial first aid is a critical component of emergency response and humanitarian assistance. It involves providing psychological support to individuals affected by crises, promoting coping mechanisms, and facilitating recovery.
- *Peer Support and Counseling:* Peer support programs, where individuals with lived experience of mental health challenges provide support to others, have shown promising results in developing nations. *Establishing peer support groups allows individuals with similar experiences to connect, share stories, and offer mutual encouragement.* Peer support helps reduce isolation, builds trust, and fosters a sense of belonging.
- *Mental Health in Schools:* Integrating psychosocial support and mental health education into school curricula can enhance emotional well-being and promote positive mental health practices among children and adolescents.
- Training and Capacity Building: Equipping local healthcare providers, community leaders, and educators with training in psychosocial support techniques empowers them to identify and address mental health challenges.
- Culturally Sensitive Approaches: Developing psychosocial support interventions that respect cultural norms, beliefs, and practices ensures that services are accessible and acceptable to the community.
- Stigma Reduction: Integrating stigma reduction campaigns within psychosocial support systems encourages open discussions about mental health, making it easier for individuals to seek help.
- Integration into Existing Services: Integrating psychosocial support into existing healthcare, education, and community services ensures a holistic approach to well-being. This approach also reduces the burden on specialized mental health services.
- Psychological First Aid: Training community members and healthcare providers in psychological first aid equip them to provide immediate support to individuals experiencing trauma or distress.

- Supportive Environments: Creating safe spaces where individuals can share their experiences, feelings, and concerns fosters a sense of belonging and reduces feelings of isolation.
- Youth and Adolescent Engagement: Developing psychosocial support programs that engage young people addresses their unique challenges, promotes resilience, and empowers them to support their peers.
- Family-Centered Approaches: Supporting families in understanding and addressing mental health challenges strengthens the family unit as a source of emotional support.
- Hotlines and Telepsychology: Creating hotlines and telepsychology services provides individuals with accessible avenues for seeking immediate support and guidance.
- Training Community Health Workers: Empowering community health workers with psychosocial support skills enhances their ability to provide comprehensive care and referral services.
- Continuous Monitoring and Evaluation: Regularly assessing the effectiveness of psychosocial support systems ensures that interventions remain relevant and impactful.
- Partnerships and Resource Mobilization: Collaborating with governmental agencies, non-governmental organizations, and international partners enhances resource allocation and knowledge-sharing for psychosocial support programs.

Conclusion: Building psychosocial support systems is critical to promoting mental well-being and building resilient communities. By focusing on community engagement, stigma reduction, culturally sensitive approaches, and integration into existing services, societies can establish comprehensive systems that address mental health challenges and provide individuals with the tools to cope and thrive. The collective effort to build strong psychosocial support systems contributes to a healthier, more connected, and resilient society capable of navigating public health challenges with greater strength and resilience [3, 4].

Integrating Mental Health into Public Health Programs

Integrating mental health into public health programs is a strategic approach to building resilient communities in developing nations. By considering mental health as an integral component of overall well-being, societies can develop more comprehensive and effective strategies for addressing health challenges. This section delves into the significance of integrating mental health into public health programs and the benefits it brings to individuals and communities [5, 6].

- *mhGAP Intervention Guide:* The World Health Organization's Mental Health Gap Action Programme (mhGAP) Intervention Guide provides evidence-based guidelines for non-specialized healthcare settings. Integrating mental health into primary healthcare services improves access to mental health care for underserved populations.

- *Task Shifting and Lay Health Workers:* Task shifting, which involves training non-specialist health workers or lay health workers, can expand the reach of mental health services. Lay health workers can provide basic mental health support, including counseling and referrals.
- *Policy and Advocacy:* Developing comprehensive mental health policies and advocating for increased funding and resources for mental health initiatives are vital for sustaining and expanding mental health services in developing nations.
- *Integration with Maternal and Child Health Programs:* Integrating mental health screening and support into maternal and child health programs enhances early detection of mental health issues and promotes the well-being of mothers and children.
- Recognizing the Nexus between Physical and Mental Health: Understanding the interconnectedness of physical and mental health is essential. Many physical health conditions have psychological implications, and mental well-being can impact physical health outcomes.
- Strengthening Health Systems: Embedding mental health within public health systems enhances their capacity to provide holistic care. This includes training healthcare providers to recognize and address mental health issues.
- Early Intervention and Prevention: Integrating mental health into primary healthcare facilitates early identification and intervention, preventing the escalation of mental health conditions.
- Maternal and Child Health Programs: Including psychosocial support and mental health services in maternal and child health programs addresses the mental well-being of both mothers and children, leading to better outcomes.
- School-Based Interventions: Integrating mental health education and support into schools promotes early awareness, equips students with coping skills, and reduces the stigma associated with mental health.
- Disaster Preparedness and Response: Ensuring that mental health support is part of disaster preparedness plans and responses helps individuals and communities recover from trauma and stress.
- Non-Communicable Disease Management: Integrating mental health support into chronic disease management programs improves overall patient outcomes and quality of life.
- Community Health Workers: Training community health workers to identify signs of mental distress and provide basic support extends mental health care to remote and underserved areas.
- Awareness Campaigns: Public health campaigns can include mental health awareness messages, promoting open dialogue and reducing stigma.

- Collaboration and Coordination: Integrating mental health requires collaboration between mental health specialists, public health officials, NGOs, and community leaders for comprehensive solutions.
- Data Collection and Monitoring: Collecting data on mental health within public health programs allows for tracking trends, evaluating interventions, and refining strategies.
- Resource Allocation: Integrating mental health into public health programs supports equitable allocation of resources for both physical and mental health services.
- Capacity Building: Training healthcare providers and community workers in mental health skills enhance their ability to provide effective support.

Conclusion: Integrating mental health into public health programs acknowledges the importance of mental well-being as a vital component of overall health. By embedding mental health support into various health initiatives, societies can create more resilient communities that are better equipped to navigate public health challenges. This comprehensive approach not only enhances individual well-being but also contributes to building a more cohesive and responsive healthcare system that serves the diverse needs of developing nations [5, 6].

Case Study 19: *Recognizing Mental Health Challenges in a Post-Conflict Nation.* It looks at 'Healing the Wounds - Mental Health in a Post-Conflict Nation.'

Introduction: In the aftermath of a prolonged civil war, many developing nations faced a significant burden of mental health challenges among their population. In one such post-conflict nation, mental health issues had become a pressing concern, affecting individuals across different age groups and communities.

Implementation: To address the mental health challenges in the post-conflict nation, a comprehensive mental health assessment and awareness campaign were initiated:

1. Mental Health Assessment: Mental health professionals conducted a nationwide mental health assessment to understand the prevalence and nature of mental health disorders among the population.

2. Community Awareness: A public awareness campaign was launched to destigmatize mental health issues and promote help-seeking behaviors. Community leaders and local influencers actively participated in spreading awareness.

3. Trauma-Informed Care: Training programs were organized for healthcare professionals, teachers, and community workers on trauma-informed care and psychosocial support.

4. Integration with Public Health Programs: Mental health services were integrated into existing public health programs to ensure access and continuity of care for individuals with mental health disorders.

Results: The mental health assessment revealed a high prevalence of mental health disorders, including post-traumatic stress disorder (PTSD), depression, and anxiety. The awareness campaign helped reduce the stigma surrounding mental health, encouraging more individuals to seek support. The integration of mental health services into public health programs improved access to care, and trauma-informed approaches facilitated the healing process for those affected by the war. Over time, there was a noticeable improvement in mental health outcomes, with more individuals receiving the support they needed to rebuild their lives after the conflict.

Case Study 20: *Building Psychosocial Support Systems for Vulnerable Youth in an Urban Slum.* It explores 'Rising Above Adversity - Empowering Youth with Psychosocial Support.'

Introduction: In urban slums of developing nations, vulnerable youth face various psychosocial challenges due to poverty, violence, and lack of opportunities. To address these issues and provide psychosocial support, a program was initiated in an urban slum to empower and uplift the youth.

Implementation: The psychosocial support program for vulnerable youth involved a range of interventions:

1. Safe Spaces: Safe spaces were established within the community to provide a supportive and nurturing environment for youth to express themselves and build positive relationships.

2. Life Skills Training: Youth were provided with life skills training, including communication, decision-making, and conflict resolution, to enhance their resilience and coping mechanisms.

3. Mentorship Programs: Mentors from the community and beyond were engaged to provide guidance and support to youth, acting as role models for personal and professional growth.

4. Counseling Services: Psychosocial counselors were available to address individual and group mental health concerns and offer therapeutic support.

Results: The psychosocial support program had a transformative impact on the vulnerable youth in the urban slum. The safe spaces provided an outlet for creative expression and emotional processing, fostering a sense of belonging and community. Life skills training empowered the youth to make informed decisions and overcome challenges. The mentorship programs enabled positive role modeling and inspired the youth to pursue education and vocational opportunities. The availability of counseling services addressed mental health issues and reduced distress among the youth. Overall, the program contributed to the upliftment of the youth, building their resilience and equipping them with the necessary skills to rise above adversity and create a brighter future.

Conclusion: These case studies underscore the importance of recognizing mental health challenges in developing nations, building psychosocial support systems, and integrating mental health into public health programs. By implementing targeted interventions, such as mental health assessments, community awareness campaigns, trauma-informed care, and psychosocial support programs, public health systems can effectively address mental health issues and support vulnerable populations in their journey toward healing and resilience. Integrating mental health into broader public health initiatives ensures a holistic approach to health and well-being, promoting the overall health and prosperity of individuals and communities in developing nations.

CONCLUSION

Addressing mental health challenges and promoting psychosocial well-being are essential components of public health in developing nations. By recognizing the unique socio-economic and cultural factors influencing mental health, building effective psychosocial support systems, and integrating mental health into public health programs, societies can create more resilient communities that thrive in the face of adversity. The collective effort to prioritize mental health contributes to improved well-being, productivity, and social cohesion in developing nations.

REFERENCES

[1]   Patel V, Araya R, Chatterjee S, *et al.* Treatment and prevention of mental disorders in low-income and middle-income countries. Lancet 2007; 370(9591): 991-1005.
[http://dx.doi.org/10.1016/S0140-6736(07)61240-9] [PMID: 17804058]

[2]   World Health Organization. Mental Health Atlas 2017. World Health Organization, 2018. Available from: https://apps.who.int/iris/handle/10665/272735

[3]   Inter-Agency Standing Committee (IASC). IASC Guidelines on Mental Health and Psychosocial Support in Emergency Settings. Inter-Agency Standing Committee, 2007. Available from: https://www.who.int/publications/i/item/iasc-guidelines-for-mental-health-and-psycho-ocial-support-in-emergency-settings

[4]   Patel V, Weiss HA, Chowdhary N, *et al.* Effectiveness of an intervention led by lay health counsellors for depressive and anxiety disorders in primary care in Goa, India (MANAS): a cluster randomised

controlled trial. Lancet 2010; 376(9758): 2086-95.
[http://dx.doi.org/10.1016/S0140-6736(10)61508-5] [PMID: 21159375]

[5]   Mental Health Gap Action Programme (mhGAP) Intervention Guide for Mental, Neurological and Substance Use Disorders in Non-Specialized Health Settings (Version 20). World Health Organization 2019.

[6]   Thornicroft G, Patel V. Including mental health among the new sustainable development goals. BMJ 2014; 349(aug20 5): g5189.
[http://dx.doi.org/10.1136/bmj.g5189] [PMID: 25145688]

CHAPTER 12

Disaster Preparedness and Resilience

Abstract: Disasters and emergencies pose significant challenges to communities, particularly in developing nations where resources may be limited. Prioritizing disaster preparedness and resilience is crucial for minimizing the impact of such events on public health and well-being. This chapter explores the importance of public health preparedness, building community resilience, and learning from past disaster responses in developing nations. By implementing proactive planning, fostering community engagement, and applying lessons learned, societies can enhance their capacity to cope with disasters effectively and protect their populations.

Keywords: Community resilience, Disaster preparedness, Developing nations, Emergencies, Public health.

INTRODUCTION

Public health preparedness is essential for mitigating the impact of natural disasters and emergencies on communities in developing nations. Strategies such as risk assessment, emergency response training, and early warning systems are critical for effective disaster management. By strengthening health systems, promoting community engagement, and ensuring access to essential services, societies can enhance their resilience and minimize the adverse effects of disasters on public health and well-being.

Building community resilience is a proactive approach to disaster preparedness that empowers communities to withstand and recover from disasters. Strategies such as strengthening social networks, empowering local leadership, and promoting knowledge and skills contribute to building resilient communities. By investing in infrastructure, promoting social cohesion, and engaging vulnerable groups, societies can create stronger and more prepared communities capable of coping with adversity.

Reflecting on past disaster responses provides valuable insights for improving future preparedness and response efforts. Lessons such as the importance of communication, community engagement, and addressing mental health needs highlight key areas for improvement. By adopting a flexible and inclusive approach, prioritizing early warning systems, and leveraging local resources, societies can enhance their resilience and minimize the impact of disasters on public health and well-being.

Public Health Preparedness for Natural Disasters and Emergencies

Public health preparedness is critical to building resilient communities in developing nations. Natural disasters and emergencies can have far-reaching impacts on public health, necessitating comprehensive planning, coordination, and response strategies. This section explores the importance of public health preparedness in the face of natural disasters and emergencies and outlines key strategies for enhancing community resilience [1, 2].

- *Disaster Risk Assessment and Planning:* Conducting comprehensive disaster risk assessments and developing robust disaster management plans are essential components of public health preparedness. Understanding the specific risks and vulnerabilities of a region enables effective allocation of resources and targeted interventions.
- *Emergency Response Training and Drills:* Providing training to healthcare workers, first responders, and community members on disaster response protocols and conducting regular drills helps enhance preparedness and coordination during actual emergencies.
- *Stockpiling and Supply Chain Management:* Maintaining strategic stockpiles of medical supplies, medicines, and emergency equipment and ensuring efficient supply chain management are crucial in addressing immediate health needs during disasters.
- Understanding Vulnerabilities: Identifying local vulnerabilities and understanding the potential health risks posed by different types of disasters are foundational steps. This knowledge guides preparedness efforts tailored to the specific risks of each community.
- Multi-Sectoral Collaboration: Effective disaster preparedness involves collaboration across sectors, including health, emergency services, government agencies, NGOs, and community organizations. Coordinated efforts ensure a cohesive response.
- Developing Contingency Plans: Creating comprehensive contingency plans that outline roles, responsibilities, and protocols for different phases of a disaster response ensures a swift and coordinated reaction.
- Strengthening Health Systems: Ensuring that healthcare facilities, clinics, and hospitals have disaster-resistant infrastructure, emergency medical supplies, and trained personnel enhances the healthcare response during emergencies.

- Early Warning Systems: Implementing effective early warning systems enables communities to receive timely alerts about impending disasters, allowing for proactive evacuation and preparation.
- Community Engagement and Training: Engaging communities in disaster preparedness education empowers individuals to respond effectively during emergencies. Training sessions can cover first aid, evacuation procedures, and disaster management.
- Safe Water and Sanitation: Ensuring access to safe water and proper sanitation facilities prevents the outbreak of waterborne diseases in the aftermath of disasters.
- Emergency Shelters and Psychosocial Support: Establishing safe and secure emergency shelters equipped with psychosocial support services addresses the physical and mental well-being of displaced individuals.
- Continuity of Essential Services: Developing strategies to maintain essential healthcare services during disasters, including maternal and child health, chronic disease management, and emergency care, is crucial.
- Coordination Centres and Communication: Establishing emergency coordination centers facilitates real-time communication and data sharing among response agencies and organizations.
- Evacuation Planning: Designing evacuation plans that consider the needs of vulnerable populations, such as the elderly, children, and individuals with disabilities, ensures their safety during emergencies.
- Post-Disaster Recovery: Planning for the post-disaster recovery phase, including rehabilitation and rebuilding, helps communities transition back to normalcy while addressing long-term health and psychosocial needs.

Conclusion: Public health preparedness for natural disasters and emergencies is essential to building resilient communities. By recognizing local vulnerabilities, collaborating across sectors, engaging communities, and establishing comprehensive response strategies, societies can effectively mitigate the impact of disasters on public health and well-being. The collective effort to prioritize disaster preparedness contributes to building communities better equipped to navigate challenges, protect their residents, and foster resilience in the face of adversity [1, 2].

Building Community Resilience to Cope with Disasters

Building community resilience is a proactive approach to disaster preparedness that empowers communities to effectively cope with and recover from the impacts of disasters. By fostering resilience, societies in developing nations can minimize the adverse effects of disasters on public health and well-being. This section delves into the strategies and considerations for building community resilience and creating stronger and more prepared communities [3, 4].

- *Strengthening Social Networks:* Strong social networks and community cohesion are vital in times of crisis. Nurturing social connections enhances mutual support and enables communities to respond collectively to challenges.
- *Empowering Local Leadership:* Empowering local leaders and involving communities in disaster planning and decision-making fosters a sense of ownership and accountability, leading to more effective disaster response. *Engaging community members in disaster preparedness planning empowers them to take an active role in their safety. Including local knowledge and perspectives ensures that strategies are contextually relevant.*
- *Promoting Knowledge and Skills:* Providing training and education on disaster preparedness, first aid, and psychosocial support equips community members with the necessary knowledge and skills to respond to emergencies.
- *Infrastructure and Environmental Resilience:* Investing in resilient infrastructure, such as flood-resistant housing and reinforced buildings, can mitigate the impact of disasters and protect lives and property.
- Education and Awareness: Raising awareness about different types of disasters, potential risks, and preventive measures equips individuals with the knowledge needed to make informed decisions during emergencies.
- Capacity Building and Training: Providing training in first aid, search and rescue, and other essential skills enables community members to respond effectively when disaster strikes.
- Social Cohesion and Networking: Promoting social connections and networking within communities fosters mutual support during crises. Strong social ties help individuals cope with stress and trauma.
- Local Resource Utilization: Utilizing local resources, skills, and knowledge enhances a community's ability to respond to disasters with limited external assistance.
- Risk Reduction Initiatives: Implementing risk reduction initiatives, such as reinforcing buildings against earthquakes or creating flood-resistant infrastructure, minimizes the impact of disasters.
- Economic Diversification: Encouraging economic diversification helps communities become less reliant on single industries or resources, reducing vulnerability to economic shocks after disasters.
- Community-Based Early Warning Systems: Establishing early warning systems at the community level allows for timely alerts and proactive responses, reducing casualties and damage.
- Psychosocial Support: Providing psychosocial support and counseling services helps individuals and communities process trauma and maintain emotional well-being.

- Cultural Preservation: Valuing and preserving cultural practices and traditions enhances a community's sense of identity and can contribute to its ability to cope during and after disasters.
- Empowering Vulnerable Groups: Paying special attention to vulnerable populations, such as the elderly, children, and people with disabilities, ensures that their specific needs are considered in disaster preparedness plans.
- Community-Based Disaster Recovery Plans: Developing community-led recovery plans allows residents to identify priorities and allocate resources for rebuilding after disasters.
- Partnerships and Collaboration: Collaborating with governmental agencies, non-governmental organizations, and local businesses strengthens the collective effort to build community resilience.
- Long-Term Planning and Sustainability: Sustaining efforts to build community resilience requires long-term planning and continued engagement to ensure that preparedness becomes an integral part of community culture.

Conclusion: Building community resilience is an investment in the future well-being of societies in developing nations. By engaging community members, fostering awareness, and equipping individuals with the necessary skills and resources, societies can create communities that are better prepared to cope with disasters and recover swiftly. The collective effort to build community resilience contributes to public health and safety, enhances social cohesion, and fosters a culture of proactive preparedness that ultimately saves lives and minimizes the impact of disasters [3, 4].

Expanding the Role of Resilient Communities in Post-Disaster Recovery

Resilient communities are those that can absorb the shock of a disaster, recover quickly, and adapt to future risks. In post-disaster contexts, community resilience is crucial in mobilizing local resources, fostering social cohesion, and ensuring sustainable recovery. This section explores how resilient communities contribute to both short-term relief efforts and long-term recovery strategies, ensuring that recovery is sustainable and builds adaptive capacity for future disasters [5].

Key Components of Community Resilience in Recovery

1. Social Capital and Collective ActionSocial networks and relationships are among the most vital resources in post-disaster recovery. Communities with strong social capital - where trust, cooperation, and reciprocity are deeply ingrained - tend to mobilize faster. Neighborhood support groups, local businesses, and faith-based organizations can help distribute resources, share information, and provide emotional support, enhancing recovery efforts.

- *Example*: After the 2010 Haiti earthquake, community-based organizations played a crucial role in organizing shelters, distributing food, and providing healthcare in the absence of formal institutions, demonstrating the value of local knowledge and collective action.

2. Community-Led Recovery Initiatives Empowering communities to lead their recovery efforts can ensure that the process reflects local priorities and needs. Engaging local stakeholders in decision-making ensures that recovery programs are more culturally appropriate and sustainable.

- *Example*: In the aftermath of Typhoon Haiyan in the Philippines, communities took charge of rebuilding efforts through local cooperatives. These cooperatives were able to rebuild homes, restore livelihoods, and establish early-warning systems that would mitigate future disaster risks.

3. Adaptive Learning and Capacity Building Disasters provide opportunities for communities to learn, adapt, and build capacities for future risk management. By incorporating lessons from past disasters, communities can adjust their strategies, update emergency preparedness plans, and improve infrastructure resilience.

- *Example*: Following Hurricane Katrina, the Lower Ninth Ward in New Orleans implemented community-driven recovery programs that focused on green infrastructure, elevating homes, and improving flood management systems. This approach not only sped up recovery but also made the area more resilient to future floods.

4. Public-Private Partnerships Post-disaster recovery can be accelerated through partnerships between local governments, NGOs, businesses, and community groups. Such collaborations can leverage resources, skills, and knowledge, ensuring that recovery initiatives are comprehensive and inclusive.

- *Example*: In Japan, following the 2011 earthquake and tsunami, public-private partnerships led to the rapid restoration of transportation infrastructure, housing, and social services. Community involvement in these partnerships helped ensure that local needs were met and recovery was more holistic.

5. Livelihood Restoration and Economic Resilience A key aspect of long-term recovery is restoring livelihoods. Communities that can quickly restart their economies and rebuild local industries are more likely to bounce back from disasters. Recovery efforts that focus on economic resilience ensure that individuals and businesses can sustain themselves post-disaster.

- *Example*: In Aceh, Indonesia, after the 2004 tsunami, local communities rebuilt their fishing industry through micro-loans and grants supported by NGOs. These efforts helped restore economic stability and provided a sustainable source of income for many families.

Long-Term Recovery Strategies for Resilient Communities

1. Inclusive Planning and ParticipationEncouraging broad participation from diverse community members—including women, youth, and marginalized groups—ensures that recovery strategies are inclusive and equitable. It strengthens social cohesion and ensures that all voices are heard in decision-making processes, which is essential for rebuilding the social fabric after a disaster.

2. Building Back BetterThe concept of "building back better" focuses on rebuilding infrastructure, homes, and services to be more resilient to future disasters. This involves upgrading building standards, integrating climate adaptation strategies, and ensuring that critical services like healthcare and education are more robust in the face of future risks.

3. Sustaining Long-Term Mental Health SupportMental health is often overlooked in post-disaster recovery, yet it plays a critical role in community resilience. Long-term mental health support systems help individuals and families cope with trauma and build the psychological resilience necessary to face future disasters.

4. Institutional Support and Policy Frameworks Governments and local authorities play a crucial role in fostering community resilience by providing institutional support, funding recovery efforts, and implementing policies that promote sustainable development. Effective policies ensure that communities receive the necessary support to recover and become more resilient.

Conclusion: Fostering Resilient Communities for Future Disasters

Incorporating resilience-building measures into post-disaster recovery is not only essential for addressing immediate needs but also for ensuring long-term sustainability. Communities that are empowered to take the lead in recovery efforts, adapt to new challenges, and foster strong social networks are better equipped to face future disasters. By prioritizing local leadership, fostering partnerships, and integrating resilience into recovery planning, communities can transform disaster recovery into an opportunity for sustainable growth and development.

This expanded section on resilient communities provides a comprehensive look at how communities can be agents of their recovery and how they can emerge stronger from the challenges posed by disasters.

Lessons Learned from Past Disaster Responses

Reflecting on past disaster responses is a crucial step in building resilient communities in developing nations. Every disaster presents opportunities to learn and improve, refining strategies for future preparedness and response efforts. This section delves into the importance of learning from past disaster responses and highlights the key lessons that can shape more effective and resilient approaches in the future [6, 7].

- *Communication and Coordination:* Effective communication and coordination among various stakeholders, including government agencies, NGOs, and international organizations, are essential for a coherent and efficient disaster response.
- *Importance of Community Engagement:* Engaging affected communities in all stages of disaster management ensures that response efforts are culturally sensitive, contextually appropriate, and responsive to local needs. *Engaging and empowering local communities in disaster responses enhance effectiveness and local ownership. Communities are often the first responders and have valuable insights into local needs.*
- *Addressing Mental Health and Psychosocial Needs*: Recognizing the mental health and psychosocial needs of disaster-affected individuals is crucial. Integrating psychosocial support into disaster response helps address the long-term effects of trauma and stress. *Past disaster responses highlight the significance of including psychosocial support in response efforts to address the mental and emotional well-being of survivors.*
- *Resilience as a Continuum:* Viewing resilience as a continuum that spans pre-disaster, during-disaster, and post-disaster phases enables a comprehensive approach to disaster management, including preparedness, response, and recovery.
- Importance of Preparedness: Disasters emphasize the necessity of proactive preparedness measures. Communities that have invested in training, early warning systems, and resource stockpiling are better equipped to respond effectively.
- Timely Communication: Effective communication is vital during disasters. Lessons from past responses underscore the need for clear and timely dissemination of information to minimize confusion and panic.

- Multi-Sectoral Collaboration: Past responses highlight the value of collaboration between government agencies, NGOs, healthcare providers, and local businesses. A coordinated approach maximizes resources and expertise.
- Flexibility and Adaptability: Disasters are unpredictable, and responses must be adaptable. Past experiences emphasize the need for flexible plans that can be adjusted based on evolving circumstances.
- Inclusion of Vulnerable Groups: Lessons from past responses stress the importance of considering the needs of vulnerable populations, including the elderly, children, and people with disabilities, in disaster planning.
- Logistical Challenges: Addressing logistical challenges, such as transportation, supply chain disruptions, and communication breakdowns, is crucial for effective response efforts.
- Early Warning Systems: Effective early warning systems that provide accurate and timely information can significantly reduce casualties and damages.
- Local Resource Utilization: Lessons from past responses underscore the importance of utilizing local resources and knowledge to complement external assistance during disasters.
- Post-Disaster Recovery: The recovery phase is as critical as the immediate response. Past experiences emphasize the need for sustained support during rebuilding to restore communities to their pre-disaster conditions or better.
- Data Collection and Documentation: Gathering data and documenting lessons learned from disaster responses facilitate informed decision-making and continuous improvement in future efforts.
- Cultural Sensitivity: Cultural norms and practices influence disaster responses. Being culturally sensitive in planning and execution ensures that interventions are well-received and effective.
- Global Collaboration and Knowledge Sharing: Disasters transcend borders. International collaboration and sharing of best practices from different regions enrich disaster preparedness and response strategies.

Conclusion: Learning from past disaster responses is essential for building resilient communities that can effectively navigate public health challenges. By analyzing successes and shortcomings, societies in developing nations can refine their strategies, enhance coordination, and implement more robust disaster preparedness measures. The collective effort to apply lessons learned contributes to building communities that are better equipped to protect their residents, minimize the impact of disasters, and foster a culture of continuous improvement in the face of adversity [6, 7].

Case Study 21: *Public Health Preparedness for Cyclones in a Coastal Community.* It looks at 'Weathering the Storm - Cyclone Preparedness in a Coastal Village.'

Introduction: Coastal communities are vulnerable to the devastating impacts of cyclones and other natural disasters. In a coastal village regularly affected by cyclones, public health preparedness plays a crucial role in mitigating the risks and protecting the community during such calamities.

Implementation: To enhance public health preparedness for cyclones, a comprehensive disaster preparedness plan was developed and implemented in the coastal village:

1. Early Warning System: An effective early warning system was established, providing timely and accurate information about approaching cyclones. Community members were trained to recognize warning signals and take appropriate actions.

2. Evacuation Plan: The community was involved in formulating a cyclone evacuation plan and identifying safe shelters and evacuation routes. Vulnerable individuals, such as the elderly and disabled, were given special attention to ensure their safety during evacuations.

3. Stockpiling Essential Supplies: Essential medical supplies, first aid kits, and clean water were stockpiled in advance to ensure immediate access during and after the cyclone.

4. Training Healthcare Workers: Healthcare professionals received specialized training in disaster response and management to provide emergency medical care during cyclones.

Results: The public health preparedness plan significantly reduced the health risks during cyclones in the coastal village. The early warning system enabled timely evacuation, minimizing casualties and injuries. The existence of safe shelters and stockpiled supplies ensured that the community's immediate needs were met during and after the cyclone. The training of healthcare workers improved the efficiency of medical response, allowing prompt and appropriate medical assistance to those in need. Overall, the preparedness measures helped the coastal village cope better with cyclones and enhanced its resilience to natural disasters.

Case Study 22: *Building Community Resilience to Flooding in a Riverine Settlement.* It looks at 'Rising Above the Floods - Building Resilience in a Riverine Community.'

Introduction: Riverine settlements are susceptible to recurrent flooding, which poses severe challenges to public health and community well-being. In a riverine settlement, building community resilience was essential to withstand the adverse impacts of seasonal flooding.

Implementation: To build resilience in the riverine settlement, a community-based disaster resilience program was launched:

1. Community-Based Disaster Committees: Community-based disaster committees were formed, comprising local leaders, volunteers, and representatives from various sectors. These committees were responsible for disaster risk reduction planning and coordination.

2. Early Warning Systems: Early warning systems were set up to monitor river levels and provide timely flood alerts to the community.

3. Community Training: Community members received training on disaster preparedness, first aid, and basic search and rescue techniques. They were also educated on safe water and sanitation practices during floods.

4. Flood-Resistant Infrastructure: Flood-resistant infrastructure, such as raised community centers and elevated houses, was constructed to minimize flood damage to essential facilities.

Results: The community-based disaster resilience program significantly improved the riverine settlement's ability to cope with flooding. The formation of disaster committees facilitated better coordination and communication during floods. The early warning systems enabled timely evacuation, reducing loss of life and property damage. Community members' training enhanced their capacity to respond effectively during emergencies. The flood-resistant infrastructure protected essential facilities, allowing a faster recovery after the floods. The riverine settlement demonstrated increased resilience and adapted better to the cyclical nature of flooding, fostering a sense of empowerment and preparedness in the face of disasters.

Conclusion: These case studies illustrate the importance of public health preparedness for natural disasters, building community resilience to cope with disasters, and learning from past disaster responses. By implementing targeted interventions, such as early warning systems, evacuation plans, community training, and flood-resistant infrastructure, public health systems can effectively respond to disasters, reduce health risks, and enhance community resilience. Drawing lessons from past disaster responses enables communities to continuously improve their preparedness and response mechanisms, fostering a culture of resilience and adaptability in the face of natural calamities.

CONCLUSION

Disaster preparedness and resilience are integral components of public health in developing nations. By implementing proactive strategies, fostering community engagement, and learning from past experiences, societies can enhance their capacity to cope with disasters effectively. The collective effort to prioritize disaster preparedness contributes to building stronger and more resilient communities capable of protecting their populations and fostering well-being in the face of adversity.

REFERENCES

[1] World Health Organization. Emergency response framework. World Health Organization, 2019. ISBN: 9789241512299. Available from: https://www.who.int/publications/i/item/9789241512299

[2] United Nations International Strategy for Disaster Reduction (UNISDR). Sendai Framework for Disaster Risk Reduction 2015-2030. United Nations International Strategy for Disaster Reduction (UNISDR), 2015. Available from: Sendai_Framework_for_Disaster_Risk_Reduction_2015-2030.pdf

[3] Norris FH, Stevens SP, Pfefferbaum B, Wyche KF, Pfefferbaum RL. Community resilience as a metaphor, theory, set of capacities, and strategy for disaster readiness. Am J Community Psychol 2008; 41(1-2): 127-50.
[http://dx.doi.org/10.1007/s10464-007-9156-6] [PMID: 18157631]

[4] Aldrich DP, Meyer MA. Social capital and community resilience. Am Behav Sci 2015; 59(2): 254-69.
[http://dx.doi.org/10.1177/0002764214550299]

[5] Aldrich DP. Building Resilience: Social Capital in Post-Disaster Recovery. University of Chicago Press 2012.
[http://dx.doi.org/10.7208/chicago/9780226012896.001.0001]

[6] World Health Organization. Inter-Agency Humanitarian Evaluation of the Response to Cyclone Idai in Mozambique. World Health Organization, 2020. Available from: https://cdn.who.int/media/docs/default-source/documents/evaluation/iahe-mozambique-summary-eng.pdf?sfvrsn=a33bebce_4

[7] Alexander DE. Resilience and disaster risk reduction: an etymological journey. Nat Hazards Earth Syst Sci 2013; 13(11): 2707-16.
[http://dx.doi.org/10.5194/nhess-13-2707-2013]

CHAPTER 13

Empowering Women and Girls in Public Health

Abstract: Empowering women and girls in public health is essential for achieving sustainable development and fostering resilient communities. Gender equity and equality are fundamental for improving health outcomes and promoting holistic well-being. By advancing gender equity in public health interventions, promoting women's health and access to healthcare, and empowering girls through education and health initiatives, societies can unlock their full potential and create healthier, more prosperous communities. This chapter explores the significance of empowering women and girls in public health and outlines strategies to achieve gender equity and promote well-being.

Keywords: Empowerment, Gender equity, Girls' education, Public health, Women's health.

INTRODUCTION

Advancing gender equity in public health interventions is crucial for building resilient communities in developing nations. Gender-responsive programming, women's participation in decision-making, and addressing gender-based violence are key strategies for promoting gender equity in public health. Ensuring equal access to healthcare services, education, and economic opportunities empowers women and girls to actively participate in their communities and improves overall well-being.

Promoting women's health and ensuring their access to quality healthcare services are essential steps toward building resilient communities. Providing gender-specific health services, addressing non-communicable diseases, and promoting sexual and reproductive health rights contribute to improved maternal and child health outcomes. Integrating women's health services into primary healthcare systems and reducing financial barriers to care enhance access and promote well-being.

Empowering girls through education and health initiatives is a transformative approach to building resilient communities. Investing in girls' education, promoting menstrual health and hygiene, and creating safe and inclusive school environments contribute to their overall well-being and empowerment. Providing girls with access to healthcare services, reproductive health education, and mental health support prepares them to make informed decisions and thrive.

Advancing Gender Equity in Public Health Interventions

Gender equity is a cornerstone of building resilient communities in developing nations. Advancing gender equity in public health interventions recognizes the unique health challenges and needs faced by women and girls. By ensuring equal access to healthcare, resources, and opportunities, societies can promote holistic well-being and empower women and girls to actively participate in their communities. This section delves into the significance of gender equity in public health interventions and outlines strategies to achieve it [1, 2].

- *Gender-Responsive Programming:* Integrating a gender perspective into public health interventions ensures that the unique needs and experiences of women and men are addressed. Gender-responsive programming promotes inclusivity and effectiveness.
- *Women's Participation in Decision-Making:* Encouraging and facilitating women's participation in health policy and decision-making processes enhances the representation of their interests and experiences in shaping public health strategies.
- *Gender Mainstreaming:* Embedding gender considerations across all levels of public health planning and implementation helps identify and address gender disparities in health outcomes and access to services.
- *Addressing Gender-Based Violence:* Tackling gender-based violence is critical in promoting women's health and well-being. Public health initiatives should include measures to prevent and respond to violence against women. *Interventions should focus on prevention, support for survivors, and changing harmful norms and attitudes.*
- Understanding Gender Dynamics: Recognizing the diverse roles, responsibilities, and vulnerabilities of women, girls, men, and boys is crucial. Gender-sensitive approaches consider the social, cultural, and economic factors that influence health outcomes.
- Equal Access to Healthcare Services: Ensuring that women and girls have the same access to healthcare services as men and boys is fundamental. This includes maternal and reproductive health services, family planning, and preventive care.
- Education and Economic Empowerment: Promoting education for girls and women empowers them to make informed health decisions, pursue economic opportunities, and contribute to community development. Supporting women's economic empowerment through income generation and entrepreneurship

opportunities not only improves financial stability but also enhances overall well-being.

- Reproductive and Maternal Health: Tailoring reproductive and maternal health programs to the specific needs of women ensures safe pregnancies, deliveries, and postpartum care.
- Family Planning and Contraception: Providing access to a range of family planning methods empowers women to make choices about their reproductive health, contributing to healthier families and communities.
- Nutrition and Food Security: Integrating gender considerations into nutrition programs acknowledges that women often play a central role in household food security and ensure their access to adequate nutrition.
- Leadership and Decision-Making: Creating spaces for women to participate in community leadership and decision-making processes ensures that their perspectives are represented in public health policies and programs.
- Data Collection and Analysis: Collecting sex-disaggregated data helps identify gender-specific health disparities, enabling targeted interventions to address them.
- Gender-Responsive Disaster Planning: Designing disaster preparedness and response plans that account for the unique needs of women and girls ensures their safety and well-being during emergencies.
- Capacity Building for Healthcare Providers: Training healthcare providers in gender-sensitive care ensures that they understand and address the specific health needs of women and girls.
- Promoting Gender Norms Change: Educational campaigns and community dialogues can challenge harmful gender norms and stereotypes, fostering a more equitable society.
- Collaboration and Partnerships: Collaborating with women's organizations, NGOs, and governmental bodies dedicated to gender equity amplifies the impact of public health interventions.

Conclusion: Advancing gender equity in public health interventions is pivotal for building resilient communities. By prioritizing women's and girls' health needs, promoting their empowerment, and addressing gender disparities, societies in developing nations can create more inclusive and healthier communities. The collective effort to advance gender equity not only improves the well-being of women and girls but also contributes to the overall social, economic, and public health progress of nations [1, 2].

Promoting Women's Health and Access to Healthcare

Promoting women's health and ensuring their access to quality healthcare services are essential steps toward building resilient communities in developing nations.

Women's health has far-reaching implications, not only for individuals but also for families and communities as a whole. This section delves into the significance of prioritizing women's health and outlines strategies to enhance their access to healthcare, contributing to improved well-being and empowerment [3, 4].

- Gender-Specific Health Services: Creating gender-specific health services that address women's unique needs, such as reproductive health, maternal care, and gynecological services, ensures comprehensive care.
- *Non-Communicable Diseases (NCDs) Prevention and Treatment:* Addressing gender-specific risk factors and barriers to healthcare access related to non-communicable diseases can improve women's overall health and quality of life.
- *Sexual and Reproductive Health Rights:* Promoting sexual and reproductive health rights empowers women to make informed choices about their bodies, including access to contraceptive methods and safe abortion services. *Empowering women with information about and access to a range of family planning methods enables them to make informed decisions about their reproductive health and family size.*
- Maternal and Reproductive Health: Offering comprehensive maternal and reproductive health services, including prenatal care, safe deliveries, and postpartum support, reduces maternal and neonatal mortality rates.
- Cervical and Breast Cancer Screening: Implementing regular screenings for cervical and breast cancer detects these diseases at early stages, increasing chances of successful treatment and survival.
- Nutrition and Anaemia Prevention: Promoting balanced nutrition and iron supplementation during pregnancy and beyond reduces the risk of anemia and its associated health complications.
- Addressing Gender-Based Violence: Ensuring that healthcare services address the physical and mental health needs of survivors of gender-based violence is essential for healing and recovery.
- Mobile Clinics and Outreach Programs: Deploying mobile clinics and outreach programs to remote or underserved areas increases women's access to healthcare services, particularly in regions with limited infrastructure.
- Health Education and Awareness: Providing health education to women about preventive measures, hygiene, nutrition, and maternal care empowers them to make informed decisions about their health.
- Training Healthcare Providers: Educating healthcare providers about gender-sensitive care and women's health needs improves the quality of care women receive.
- Antenatal and Postnatal Care: Ensuring that antenatal and postnatal care services are available, accessible, and culturally sensitive supports women's well-being during pregnancy and after childbirth.

- Integration with Primary Healthcare: Integrating women's health services into primary healthcare systems ensures that women can access care as part of their overall health needs.
- Community Health Workers: Training community health workers, especially women, to provide basic healthcare services enhances access to care in remote areas.
- Financial Accessibility: Reducing financial barriers to healthcare through subsidized services or health insurance schemes ensures that women can access care regardless of their economic status.
- Engaging Men and Communities: Involving men and communities in discussions about women's health promotes supportive environments and encourages men to participate in women's health decisions.

Conclusion: Promoting women's health and ensuring their access to healthcare services is a crucial step in building resilient communities. By recognizing and addressing the unique health needs of women, societies in developing nations can empower women, improve maternal and child health outcomes, and create healthier families and communities. The collective effort to prioritize women's health and access to healthcare contributes to overall community well-being, social development, and the building of resilient societies capable of navigating public health challenges with strength and equity [3, 4].

Sexual Violence and Crimes Against Women: A Public Health Crisis

Sexual violence and crimes against women are pervasive issues that affect the physical, psychological, and social well-being of women and girls globally. These forms of violence are not only violations of human rights but also pose significant public health challenges. They contribute to a wide range of health problems, including physical injuries, sexually transmitted infections (STIs), unintended pregnancies, mental health disorders, and long-term trauma [5, 6].

The Prevalence and Impact of Sexual Violence

Sexual violence, which includes rape, sexual assault, and coercion, occurs across all societies, but women and girls in marginalized or vulnerable situations, such as in conflict zones, refugee camps, or impoverished communities, face heightened risks. Globally, it is estimated that one in three women experiences physical or sexual violence in her lifetime, often at the hands of an intimate partner. In some regions, this figure is even higher due to cultural norms that tolerate or justify violence against women.

The impact of sexual violence extends beyond the immediate physical harm. Survivors often face stigma, social exclusion, and a lack of access to appropriate healthcare services, which can exacerbate their trauma. Many may not report their experiences due to fear of retribution, shame, or mistrust in legal systems. This underreporting means that the true scale of sexual violence is often underestimated.

Public Health Consequences of Sexual Violence

The health consequences of sexual violence are vast and intersect with other public health challenges:

- **Physical Health:** Survivors may suffer from acute injuries, chronic pain, and sexual and reproductive health complications such as STIs, including HIV. They are also at increased risk of unsafe abortions and maternal mortality.
- **Mental Health:** Depression, anxiety, post-traumatic stress disorder (PTSD), and suicidal tendencies are common among survivors. The psychological toll can last for years, affecting not only the survivors but also their families and communities.
- **Economic Impact:** Sexual violence can lead to loss of employment or educational opportunities, further entrenching poverty and economic dependence, especially in societies where women already face systemic disadvantages.

The Role of Public Health Systems in Addressing Sexual Violence

Public health systems play a crucial role in addressing the aftermath of sexual violence and preventing future occurrences. This requires a multi-faceted approach that includes:

- **Access to Comprehensive Healthcare:** Survivors need access to timely medical care, including emergency contraception, post-exposure prophylaxis (PEP) for HIV, STI testing, and mental health services. Sexual violence response services should be integrated into primary healthcare and maternal health services to ensure that women and girls receive the care they need without facing stigma or discrimination.
- **Legal and Social Support:** Public health institutions should work in tandem with legal systems to ensure that survivors have access to justice. This includes providing forensic examinations and expert testimonies and ensuring that health services are survivor-centered and respectful of confidentiality.
- **Community-Based Interventions:** Public health initiatives should engage communities in changing attitudes towards sexual violence and dismantling harmful gender norms. Education and advocacy efforts are essential to prevent violence and encourage survivors to seek help. Empowering women and girls

through education and economic opportunities can also reduce their vulnerability to violence.

Preventing Sexual Violence through Public Health Interventions

Prevention is a key aspect of reducing sexual violence and its impact on women's health. Public health strategies should focus on:

- **Education and Awareness Campaigns:** Raising awareness about consent, gender equality, and the consequences of sexual violence can shift societal norms and reduce tolerance for violence against women. School-based programs that educate boys and girls about healthy relationships, respect, and consent are vital in changing future behaviors.
- **Support for Survivors of Violence:** Ensuring that women and girls who have experienced sexual violence have access to comprehensive services, including shelters, legal aid, and mental health counseling, is crucial. The creation of survivor support networks can foster a sense of solidarity and empowerment.
- **Engaging Men and Boys:** Prevention programs that involve men and boys in discussions about masculinity, respect, and non-violence are critical in reducing the prevalence of sexual violence. Public health initiatives that promote positive male role models and challenge toxic masculinity can contribute to cultural change.

Intersectionality and Vulnerability

It is important to recognize the intersectionality of sexual violence, where factors such as race, socioeconomic status, disability, and sexual orientation can exacerbate vulnerabilities. For example, women from ethnic minorities, refugees, or women with disabilities often face compounded risks of violence and discrimination. Public health interventions must be tailored to address the unique needs of these groups, ensuring that no one is left behind.

Conclusion: Addressing sexual violence and crimes against women is fundamental to improving the health and well-being of women and girls. By tackling the root causes of gender-based violence, strengthening healthcare systems, and fostering a culture of zero tolerance towards violence, public health initiatives can empower women and girls to live free from fear and harm. Sexual violence is not only a public health issue but a societal one, requiring collective action from governments, healthcare providers, communities, and individuals.

Empowering Girls through Education and Health Initiatives

Empowering girls through education and health initiatives is a pivotal step toward building resilient communities in developing nations. By investing in girls' education and ensuring their access to quality healthcare, societies can break cycles of poverty, promote gender equity, and improve overall well-being. This section explores the transformative impact of empowering girls through education and health initiatives and outlines strategies to achieve these goals [7, 8].

- *Girls' Education and Health Literacy: Ensuring that girls have equal access to quality education opportunities fosters their cognitive, social, and economic development. Education is a powerful tool for breaking intergenerational cycles of poverty.* Investing in girls' education and health literacy equips them with the knowledge and skills to make informed decisions about their health and well-being. *Designing a curriculum that challenges gender stereotypes and promotes positive gender norms creates an inclusive learning environment that empowers girls.*
- *Adolescent Sexual and Reproductive Health:* Addressing the specific sexual and reproductive health needs of adolescent girls promotes safe practices and reduces the risks of early pregnancies and related health issues.
- *Nutrition and Hygiene:* Implementing nutrition and hygiene programs targeted at girls enhances their overall health and reduces the prevalence of malnutrition and related diseases.
- *Gender Norms and Social Empowerment:* Challenging harmful gender norms and promoting girls' social empowerment contribute to creating an enabling environment for their holistic development.
- Promoting School Enrollment and Retention: Implementing measures to encourage girls' school enrollment and retention, such as providing scholarships, menstrual hygiene support, and safe transportation, promotes equal educational opportunities.
- Health Education: Integrating health education into the curriculum equips girls with knowledge about nutrition, hygiene, reproductive health, and mental well-being.
- Life Skills Education: Teaching life skills, such as critical thinking, decision-making, communication, and problem-solving, prepares girls to navigate challenges and make informed choices.
- Menstrual Health and Hygiene Initiatives: Implementing menstrual health and hygiene initiatives, including providing sanitary products and menstrual education, ensures that girls can attend school without interruption.
- Safe and Inclusive School Spaces: Creating safe and inclusive school environments, free from gender-based violence and discrimination, enhances girls' sense of security and belonging.

- Peer Support and Mentorship: Establishing peer support groups and mentorship programs connects girls with positive role models, building their confidence and self-esteem.
- Early Childhood Development: Investing in early childhood development programs prepares girls for school by promoting cognitive, emotional, and physical development.
- Parent and Community Engagement: Engaging parents and communities in girls' education fosters support for girls' schooling, challenges traditional gender norms, and reinforces the importance of education.
- Healthcare Access and Services: Ensuring that girls have access to regular healthcare check-ups, vaccinations, and preventive care contributes to their overall well-being.
- Reproductive Health and Family Planning: Providing girls with information about reproductive health and family planning empowers them to make informed decisions about their bodies and future.
- Mental Health and Well-Being: Addressing mental health needs through awareness campaigns, counseling services, and stress management techniques supports girls' emotional well-being.
- Community Empowerment and Advocacy: Engaging communities in advocating for girls' education and health initiatives creates a supportive environment for girls' empowerment.

Conclusion: Empowering girls through education and health initiatives is a transformative approach that builds resilient communities. By investing in their education, health, and overall well-being, societies in developing nations can break down barriers, challenge gender disparities, and create a foundation for equitable development. The collective effort to empower girls improves their prospects. It enhances the social fabric and resilience of communities, fostering a future where girls can contribute positively to the advancement of their families, communities, and nations [7, 8].

Case Study 23: *Advancing Gender Equity in Maternal Health Programs in a Developing Country.* It looks at 'Breaking Barriers - Advancing Gender Equity in Maternal Health.'

Introduction: Gender disparities in maternal health are a common concern in many developing countries. In one such country, maternal mortality rates were alarmingly high, indicating significant gaps in access to quality maternal healthcare services.

Implementation: To address gender disparities in maternal health, a gender equity-focused maternal health program was implemented:

1. Access to Maternal Healthcare: The program ensured equitable access to maternal healthcare services by removing financial barriers and providing transportation support for pregnant women to access healthcare facilities.

2. Training Healthcare Professionals: Healthcare professionals received gender-sensitive training, ensuring that women were treated with dignity and respectand without discrimination during childbirth and prenatal care.

3. Community Awareness: Community awareness campaigns were launched to challenge gender norms and promote women's decision-making power in matters related to their health and pregnancy.

4. Empowerment Initiatives: Women's empowerment initiatives were integrated into maternal health programs, providing opportunities for skill-building and income-generating activities.

Results: The gender equity-focused maternal health program led to significant improvements in maternal health outcomes. The removal of financial barriers and transportation support increased the number of institutional deliveries, reducing home births and improving maternal and neonatal health. The gender-sensitive training of healthcare professionals improved the quality of care and enhanced women's experience during childbirth. The community awareness campaigns challenged gender norms, encouraging women's empowerment and involvement in maternal healthcare decision-making. The integration of empowerment initiatives contributed to women's economic independence and improved overall health and well-being. As a result, maternal mortality rates decreased, and women's health and agency in public health decisions improved.

Case Study 24: *Empowering Girls through Comprehensive Health and Education Initiatives.* It looks at 'Rising Strong - Empowering Girls for a Brighter Future.'

Introduction: In underserved communities, girls often face multiple barriers to education and healthcare, limiting their opportunities for personal development and well-being. In one such community, a comprehensive health and education initiative was launched to empower girls and support their overall growth.

Implementation: The comprehensive health and education initiative involved a multi-faceted approach to empower girls:

1. Girls' Education Programs: The initiative supported girls' education through scholarships, school infrastructure improvement, and the provision of learning materials.

2. Menstrual Health Support: Menstrual health education and hygiene supplies were provided to ensure that girls could attend school regularly and without disruption.

3. Health and Life Skills Education: Girls received health education, including reproductive health and hygiene, along with life skills training to build their confidence and decision-making abilities.

4. Safe Spaces: Safe spaces were created for girls to engage in extracurricular activities, peer support, and discussions on issues affecting their well-being.

Results: The comprehensive health and education initiative had a transformative impact on the girls in the community. The support for girls' education increased school enrollment and retention rates, providing them with opportunities for personal and professional growth. The provision of menstrual health support enabled girls to manage their menstrual hygiene with dignity, reducing absenteeism and dropout rates. Health and life skills education improved their understanding of health issues and empowered them to make informed decisions. The safe spaces provided a supportive environment for girls to express themselves, build self-esteem, and advocate for their rights. As a result, girls in the community demonstrated improved confidence, well-being, and aspirations for a brighter future.

Conclusion: These case studies highlight the significance of advancing gender equity in public health interventions, promoting women's health and access to healthcare, and empowering girls through education and health initiatives. By implementing targeted interventions, such as gender-sensitive healthcare services, women's empowerment initiatives, and girls' education programs, public health systems can promote gender equity and improve the health and well-being of women and girls in developing nations. Empowering women and girls not only enhances their own lives but also has a positive ripple effect on families, communities, and societies as a whole, contributing to more inclusive and resilient public health outcomes.

CONCLUSION

Empowering women and girls in public health is a strategic investment in sustainable development and resilient communities. By advancing gender equity, promoting women's health and access to healthcare, and empowering girls through education and health initiatives, societies can create inclusive and prosperous futures. The collective effort to prioritize gender equality and promote well-being contributes to healthier, more resilient communities capable of addressing public health challenges with strength and equity.

REFERENCES

[1]   United Nations. Transforming Our World: The 2030 Agenda for Sustainable Development. United Nations, 2015. Available from: https://sustainabledevelopment.un.org/post2015/transformingourworld

[2]   World Health Organization. Gender, Equity, and Human Rights: Health inequality monitoring. World Health Organization 2019. Available from: https://apps.who.int/iris/bitstream/handle/10665/325057/WHO-FWC-GER-17.1-eng.pdf?ua=1

[3]   World Health Organization. Women's health fact sheet. World Health Organization, 2022. Available from: https://www.who.int/health-topics/women-s-health

[4]   United Nations Population Fund (UNFPA). State of World Population 2021. United Nations Population Fund (UNFPA), 2021. Available from: https://www.unfpa.org/swop

[5]   Sardinha L, Maheu-Giroux M, Stöckl H, Meyer SR, García-Moreno C. Global, regional, and national prevalence estimates of physical or sexual, or both, intimate partner violence against women in 2018. Lancet. 2022399(10327): 803-813.
        [http://dx.doi.org/10.1016/S0140-6736(21)02664-7]

[6]   Basile KC, DeGue S, Jones K, *et al.* Sexual Violence Prevention Resource for Action: A Compilation of the Best Available Evidence. Atlanta, GA: National Center for Injury Prevention and Control, Centers for Disease Control and Prevention 2016.

[7]   UNESCO. Global Education Monitoring Report 2020. UNESCO, 2021. Available from: https://en.unesco.org/gem-report/report/2020/inclusion

[8]   United Nations Children's Fund (UNICEF). The State of the World's Children 2023. United Nations Children's Fund (UNICEF), 2023. Available from: https://www.unicef.org/reports/state-world--children-2023

CHAPTER 14

Innovative Technologies for Public Health

Abstract: Technology and innovation play a crucial role in transforming public health practices and improving health outcomes globally. Integrating technology into public health solutions, implementing mobile health (mHealth) and electronic health (eHealth) initiatives, and leveraging digital tools for data collection and analysis are key strategies for enhancing resilience and well-being in communities. By harnessing the power of technology, public health systems can become more efficient, responsive, and inclusive, ultimately leading to healthier populations and stronger communities. This chapter explores the significance of technology and innovation in public health and outlines strategies for effectively utilizing digital solutions to address health challenges and foster resilience.

Keywords: Digital tools, Data collection, Data analysis, eHealth, Innovation, mHealth, Public health, Technology.

INTRODUCTION

Technology catalyzes transforming public health practices, particularly in developing nations. Health information systems, telemedicine, mobile health solutions, and artificial intelligence are among the innovative technologies revolutionizing healthcare access and delivery. By embracing technology, public health systems can streamline processes, improve data management, and enhance decision-making, ultimately strengthening community resilience.

Mobile Health (mHealth) and eHealth initiatives leverage mobile phones and online platforms to revolutionize healthcare access and delivery. These initiatives promote health promotion, remote patient monitoring, telemedicine consultations, and health information dissemination. By harnessing mobile technology and online platforms, communities can overcome barriers to healthcare access, empower individuals with information, and enhance community well-being.

Digital tools have revolutionized data collection and analysis in public health, enabling more accurate, timely, and comprehensive insights. Mobile data collection apps, GIS technology, electronic health records, and big data analytics are among the digital tools transforming public health surveillance and decision-making. By harnessing digital tools, societies can gather and analyze health information with greater efficiency, accuracy, and speed, empowering communities to make informed decisions and respond effectively to health challenges.

Harnessing Technology for Public Health Solutions

Technology and innovation have revolutionized public health practices in developing nations. By harnessing the power of technology, communities can access information, services, and solutions that enhance their resilience and well-being. This section delves into the significance of technology in public health and outlines strategies for effectively utilizing technology to address health challenges and create resilient communities [1, 2].

- *Health Information Systems: Implementing electronic health records, data collection tools, and health information systems streamlines data management, enabling real-time monitoring and informed decision-making.* Digital health information systems streamline patient data management, allowing healthcare providers to access and share information efficiently and securely.
- *Telemedicine, Telehealth, and Virtual Care: Utilizing telemedicine platforms and virtual care services enables remote consultations, diagnoses, and treatment, particularly in underserved or remote areas.* Telemedicine and telehealth technologies enable remote medical consultations and healthcare services, improving access to healthcare, especially in remote or underserved areas.
- Mobile Health (mHealth) Solutions: Leveraging mobile phones for health communication, appointment reminders, medication adherence, and health education increases access to vital information.
- *Artificial Intelligence (AI) in Disease Detection:* AI-powered tools, such as machine learning algorithms, can analyze large datasets to detect patterns and identify disease outbreaks early, enabling prompt interventions.
- Epidemiological Surveillance: Advanced data analytics and modeling tools allow for the timely detection and monitoring of disease outbreaks, enabling proactive interventions.
- Digital Health Apps: Developing user-friendly mobile applications for health education, symptom tracking, and self-care empowers individuals to take charge of their health.
- Healthcare Supply Chain Management: Implementing technology-driven supply chain solutions enhances the efficient distribution of medical supplies and reduces stockouts.

- Remote Monitoring Devices: Using wearable devices and sensors for remote monitoring of vital signs, chronic conditions, and maternal health improves early detection and management.
- Geographical Information Systems (GIS): GIS technology helps map disease trends, identify high-risk areas, and optimize resource allocation during emergencies.
- Health Education and Awareness Campaigns: Leveraging social media, websites, and online platforms for health education campaigns disseminates accurate information and reduces misinformation.
- Data Analytics for Decision-Making: Harnessing data analytics and artificial intelligence supports evidence-based decision-making, resource allocation, and policy formulation.
- Disaster Preparedness and Early Warning Systems: Incorporating technology into disaster preparedness plans and early warning systems enhances response times and saves lives during emergencies.
- Capacity Building and Training: Online training platforms and e-learning initiatives enhance the skills of healthcare workers and community health volunteers.
- Remote Training and Consultations: Using video conferencing and online platforms, healthcare providers can receive training and consultations from experts, even in remote areas.
- Partnerships and Collaborations: Collaborating with tech companies, universities, and research institutions fosters the development of innovative public health solutions.

Conclusion: Harnessing technology for public health solutions is a dynamic strategy that empowers communities and enhances resilience. By integrating technology into public health practices, societies in developing nations can bridge gaps in healthcare access, improve information dissemination, and respond more effectively to health challenges. The collective effort to embrace technology and innovation contributes to building resilient communities capable of adapting to evolving health needs and harnessing the power of digital solutions to create a healthier and more connected future.

Mobile Health (mHealth) and eHealth Initiatives

Mobile Health (mHealth) and Electronic Health (eHealth) initiatives have emerged as game-changers in public health, particularly in developing nations. These technologies leverage the ubiquity of mobile phones and the internet to revolutionize healthcare access, empower individuals, and enhance community resilience. This section explores the significance of mHealth and eHealth initiatives and outlines strategies for effectively integrating these technologies into public health practices [3, 4].

- *mHealth Applications for Health Promotion:* mHealth applications deliver health-related information, behavior change interventions, and reminders to individuals' mobile devices, empowering them to make informed decisions about their health.
- *Remote Patient Monitoring (RPM) through mHealth:* RPM *via* mobile devices enables real-time monitoring of patients with chronic conditions, facilitating timely interventions and reducing hospitalizations.
- *eHealth Platforms for Access to Health Services:* eHealth platforms, including telemedicine portals and online appointment systems, enhance access to healthcare services, particularly for rural and marginalized communities.
- *SMS-Based Health Programs:* SMS-based health programs deliver health messages, appointment reminders, and follow-up care instructions to individuals with limited internet access, bridging the digital divide.
- Enhanced Healthcare Access: mHealth and eHealth initiatives bridge geographical gaps, enabling individuals in remote or underserved areas to access healthcare information and services.
- Health Information Dissemination: Using mobile apps, SMS, and online platforms, mHealth and eHealth initiatives deliver accurate health information, preventive measures, and treatment guidelines to a wider audience.
- Appointment Reminders and Follow-ups: Automated appointment reminders and follow-up messages *via* mobile phones reduce missed appointments and improve continuity of care.
- Telemedicine Consultations: Virtual consultations through video calls or chat platforms allow healthcare providers to diagnose and treat patients remotely, especially in areas with limited access to medical facilities.
- Medication Adherence Support: mHealth Solutions sends medication reminders and educational messages, enhancing adherence to treatment regimens for chronic conditions.
- Maternal and Child Health Support: eHealth platforms guide maternal care, pregnancy tracking, and infant health, ensuring safe pregnancies and healthy newborns.
- Monitoring Chronic Conditions: Wearable devices and smartphone apps enable individuals to monitor chronic conditions, such as diabetes or hypertension, and share data with healthcare providers.
- Disease Surveillance and Reporting: Using mobile data collection tools, health workers can report disease outbreaks, monitor trends, and respond swiftly to emerging health threats.

- Remote Training and Capacity Building: eLearning platforms offer healthcare workers and community volunteers access to training and skill development, improving the quality of care.
- Health Records and Data Management: eHealth systems digitize patient records, streamlining data management and improving the accuracy of medical histories.
- Behavioral Change Interventions: mHealth apps can promote healthy behaviors by sending reminders for exercise, nutrition, and lifestyle modifications.
- Emergency Response and Disaster Preparedness: mHealth platforms provide emergency information, alert notifications, and evacuation instructions during disasters.
- Community Engagement and Feedback: Online forums and social media platforms facilitate community engagement, allowing individuals to share health concerns, ask questions, and provide feedback.
- Partnerships and Collaboration: Collaborating with mobile network operators, tech companies, and health organizations enhances the development and reach of mHealth and eHealth initiatives.

Conclusion: mHealth and eHealth initiatives hold immense potential for transforming public health practices and building resilient communities. By leveraging mobile technology and online platforms, societies in developing nations can overcome barriers to healthcare access, empower individuals with information, and enhance community well-being. The collective effort to embrace mHealth and eHealth contributes to creating a more connected, informed, and resilient society capable of navigating public health challenges with innovation and effectiveness.

Digital Tools for Data Collection and Analysis

Digital tools have revolutionized data collection and analysis in public health, enabling more accurate, timely, and comprehensive insights. By harnessing technology, communities can gather essential health information, track trends, and make informed decisions to strengthen resilience. This section highlights the significance of digital tools for data collection and analysis and outlines strategies for leveraging technology to enhance public health efforts [5, 6].

- Mobile Data Collection Apps: Mobile apps allow health workers and field personnel to collect data directly from the field, improving accuracy and efficiency.
- Online Surveys and Questionnaires: Web-based surveys and questionnaires facilitate data collection from a wide audience, providing insights into health behaviors, concerns, and needs.

- *Geographical Information Systems (GIS): GIS technology maps disease patterns, identifies high-risk areas, and informs resource allocation during emergencies.* GIS technology visualizes and analyzes health data on maps, helping identify disease patterns, hotspots, and vulnerable populations for targeted interventions.
- *Electronic Health Records (EHRs): EHRs streamline patient data management, enabling healthcare providers to access comprehensive health histories for informed decision-making.* EHRs store patients' medical histories, diagnoses, medications, and test results electronically, improving care coordination and facilitating evidence-based decision-making.
- *Real-time Monitoring and Surveillance: Digital tools enable real-time monitoring of disease outbreaks, health indicators, and trends, allowing for swift response and intervention.* Digital surveillance systems collect and analyze health data in real time, enabling prompt detection and response to disease outbreaks and public health emergencies.
- *Wearable Devices and Sensors: Wearable health devices track vital signs, activity levels, and chronic conditions, generating data for personalized care plans.* Wearable devices, like fitness trackers and smartwatches, monitor individuals' health metrics, promoting preventive healthcare behaviors and personalized health management.
- *Big Data and Predictive Analytics: Analyzing large datasets with advanced analytics tools reveals insights about health trends, disease prevalence, and population dynamics.* Big data analytics leverage large datasets to predict disease trends, optimize healthcare resource allocation, and inform public health policies.
- Machine Learning and AI: Machine learning algorithms can predict disease outbreaks, identify high-risk populations, and optimize resource allocation.
- Data Visualization: Creating visual representations of health data, such as graphs and maps, enhances communication and understanding of complex information.
- Remote Monitoring and Telehealth: Remote monitoring devices and telehealth platforms generate data on patients' health status, supporting virtual consultations and care management.
- Surveillance of Public Health Interventions: Digital tools track the impact of public health interventions, enabling assessment of effectiveness and necessary adjustments.
- Disease Registry Systems: Digital registries compile data on specific diseases, improving tracking, treatment, and long-term management.
- Data Sharing and Collaboration: Digital platforms facilitate data sharing and collaboration between healthcare providers, researchers, and policymakers for more informed decision-making.

- Privacy and Data Security: Ensuring data security and protecting individuals' privacy are paramount in digital data collection and storage.

Conclusion: Digital tools for data collection and analysis have transformed the landscape of public health in developing nations. By harnessing technology, societies can gather and analyze health information with greater efficiency, accuracy, and speed. The utilization of digital tools empowers communities to make informed decisions, track health trends, and respond effectively to public health challenges. The collective effort to embrace digital innovations contributes to building resilient communities that can proactively address health issues and enhance overall well-being through data-driven insights and interventions.

Case Study 25: *Harnessing Technology for Disease Surveillance in a Remote Region.* It looks at 'Connecting the Dots - Technology-Driven Disease Surveillance.'

Introduction: In remote regions with limited access to healthcare facilities, disease surveillance and early detection of outbreaks pose significant challenges. In one such remote region, technology-driven disease surveillance was implemented to enhance public health monitoring and response.

Implementation: To improve disease surveillance and response, a technology-driven system was put in place:

1. Mobile Data Collection: Community health workers used mobile devices equipped with data collection applications to record health-related information during their visits to households.

2. Real-Time Data Transmission: The collected data were transmitted in real-time to a central database, enabling health authorities to access and analyze information promptly.

3. Early Warning Algorithms: The system integrated early warning algorithms, allowing for the detection of unusual health trends and potential disease outbreaks.

4. Targeted Interventions: Health authorities used the data analysis to deploy targeted interventions and resources to mitigate the impact of emerging health threats.

Results: The technology-driven disease surveillance system revolutionized public health monitoring in the remote region. Real-time data transmission improved the speed and accuracy of disease reporting, allowing for timely responses. Early warning algorithms successfully detected and contained outbreaks, preventing further transmission of infectious diseases. The targeted interventions based on data analysis effectively addressed health challenges specific to the region, leading to improved health outcomes and reduced disease burden. Overall, the technology-driven approach played a crucial role in strengthening the region's public health capacity and preparedness for emerging health threats.

Case Study 26: *Mobile Health (mHealth) Initiatives for Maternal and Child Health in an Underserved Area.* It explores 'Empowering Mothers and Improving Child Health through mHealth.'

Introduction: In underserved areas, maternal and child health outcomes often suffer due to limited access to healthcare services. To bridge this gap and improve maternal and child health, mobile health (mHealth) initiatives were implemented.

Implementation: The mHealth initiatives targeted maternal and child health through several interventions:

1. Maternal Health Messages: Pregnant women and new mothers received personalized health messages through mobile applications, providing them with information on prenatal care, nutrition, and postnatal support.

2. Child Health Tracking: Parents or caregivers used mobile apps to track their child's growth, vaccinations, and developmental milestones, receiving reminders for immunizations and health check-ups.

3. Teleconsultations: Remote communities were provided access to teleconsultations with healthcare professionals through mobile devices, enabling timely medical advice and follow-up care.

4. Data-Driven Decision-Making: Data collected through mHealth applications were analyzed to identify health trends and guide resource allocation for maternal and child health services.

Results: The mHealth initiatives led to notable improvements in maternal and child health in the underserved area. Maternal health messages increased awareness about healthy practices during pregnancy and postpartum, leading to better maternal outcomes. Child health tracking empowered parents to actively participate in their child's health and receive timely vaccinations and medical attention. Teleconsultations reduced the barriers to accessing healthcare services, ensuring prompt medical advice and care for remote communities. The data-driven approach facilitated evidence-based decision-making, optimizing resource allocation and strengthening maternal and child health services. As a result, maternal mortality rates decreased, child immunization rates improved, and overall, child health indicators showed positive trends.

Conclusion: These case studies highlight the transformative potential of harnessing technology for public health solutions, implementing mobile health (mHealth) and eHealth initiatives, and utilizing digital tools for data collection and analysis. By leveraging technology and innovation, public health systems can improve disease surveillance, enhance access to healthcare, and strengthen maternal and child health services. The adoption of technology-driven approaches fosters more efficient, data-driven decision-making, ultimately leading to improved health outcomes and better public health preparedness in developing nations.

CONCLUSION

Technology and innovation hold immense potential for transforming public health practices and building resilient communities. By harnessing the power of technology, public health systems can bridge gaps in healthcare access, improve information dissemination, and respond more effectively to health challenges. The collective effort to embrace technology and innovation contributes to creating a healthier, more connected, and resilient society capable of navigating public health challenges with innovation and effectiveness.

REFERENCES

[1]   World Health Organization. Digital Health. World Health Organization, 2021. Available from: https://www.who.int/westernpacific/health-topics/digital-health

[2]   World Health Organization. Global strategy on digital health 2020-2025. World Health Organization, 2021. Available from: https://apps.who.int/iris/handle/10665/344249

[3]   Free C, Phillips G, Galli L, *et al.* The effectiveness of mobile-health technology-based health behaviour change or disease management interventions for health care consumers: a systematic review. PLoS Med 2013; 10(1): e1001362.
[http://dx.doi.org/10.1371/journal.pmed.1001362] [PMID: 23349621]

[4]   Mechael PN. The case for mHealth in developing countries. Innov (Camb, Mass) 2009; 4(1): 103-18.
[http://dx.doi.org/10.1162/itgg.2009.4.1.103]

[5]   World Health Organization. Digital tools for COVID-19 contact tracing: operational guidance for national and subnational public health authorities. World Health Organization, 2021. Available from: https://apps.who.int/iris/handle/10665/341241

[6]   Al-Shorbaji N. Improving Healthcare Access through Digital Health: The Use of Information and Communication Technologies. IntechOpen 2022.
[http://dx.doi.org/10.5772/intechopen.99607]

CHAPTER 15

Strengthening Health Systems and Governance

Abstract: A robust health system is essential for effective public health responses and achieving universal health coverage. Strengthening health systems and governance involves enhancing leadership, building healthcare capacity, and overcoming various challenges. By prioritizing these aspects, societies can improve health outcomes, promote equity, and ensure access to quality healthcare services. This chapter explores the importance of enhancing healthcare governance and leadership, capacity building for healthcare professionals, and strategies for overcoming challenges in health system strengthening.

Keywords: Capacity building, Challenges, Governance, Health systems, Leadership, Solutions.

INTRODUCTION

Effective governance and leadership are crucial for building resilient health systems. Establishing clear governance structures, promoting multi-sectoral collaboration, and ensuring transparency and accountability are key strategies. By prioritizing inclusive decision-making and stakeholder engagement, countries can strengthen their healthcare systems and improve health outcomes.

Investing in the continuous development of healthcare professionals is essential for building resilient health systems. Strategies include fostering a culture of continuous learning, strengthening primary healthcare, and providing inclusive education and training opportunities. By equipping healthcare workers with the necessary skills and knowledge, communities can access higher-quality care and better respond to public health challenges.

Building resilient health systems involves addressing various challenges, including limited resources, health workforce shortages, and infrastructure gaps. Solutions include innovative financing mechanisms, workforce planning, and investment in infrastructure development. By adopting a multi-faceted approach and engaging with diverse stakeholders, countries can overcome these challenges and build stronger, more equitable health systems.

Enhancing Healthcare Governance and Leadership

Effective healthcare governance and leadership are foundational elements for building resilient communities and robust health systems in developing nations. Strong leadership ensures strategic decision-making, resource allocation, and coordination of efforts to address public health challenges. This section delves into the significance of enhancing healthcare governance and leadership and outlines strategies for achieving effective governance structures [1, 2].

- *Effective Governance Structures:* Establishing strong governance structures with clear roles and responsibilities is vital for ensuring accountability, transparency, and coordination within the health system.
- *Leadership Development:* Investing in leadership development programs for healthcare leaders fosters effective decision-making and strategic planning, driving positive changes in health services delivery.
- *Multi-Sectoral Collaboration:* Promoting collaboration between health and other sectors, such as education, finance, and social services, can address the social determinants of health and enhance overall population well-being.
- *Stakeholder Engagement:* Engaging stakeholders, including communities, civil society, and private sector partners, in health policy development and implementation fosters ownership and responsiveness to local needs.
- Transparent and Accountable Governance: Transparency and accountability in healthcare governance foster trust and confidence among stakeholders, promoting effective decision-making and resource utilization.
- Strong Leadership at All Levels: Leadership should extend from national to community levels, with well-trained and empowered leaders who guide policy implementation and community engagement.
- Inclusive Decision-Making: Involving diverse stakeholders, including communities, healthcare providers, policymakers, and civil society, in decision-making enhances the relevance and effectiveness of health policies.
- Policy Formulation and Implementation: Strong governance ensures that health policies are evidence-based, context-specific, and implemented efficiently to address the needs of the population.
- Regulatory Frameworks: Establishing and enforcing regulatory frameworks for healthcare services, quality standards, and professional ethics ensures the safety and well-being of patients.
- Health Workforce Development: Effective governance prioritizes the training, motivation, and equitable distribution of healthcare workers, addressing shortages and skill gaps.
- Resource Allocation and Management: Leadership ensures equitable allocation and efficient management of healthcare resources, optimizing service delivery and reducing wastage.

- Health Information Systems: Governance supports the development and maintenance of robust health information systems for data collection, analysis, and informed decision-making.

- Stakeholder Collaboration: Effective governance encourages collaboration between government bodies, NGOs, the private sector, and international partners to leverage collective expertise and resources.
- Community Engagement and Participation: Leadership actively involves communities in healthcare planning, implementation, and monitoring, ensuring that services meet local needs.
- Monitoring and Evaluation: Governance includes mechanisms for continuous monitoring and evaluation of health programs, enabling timely adjustments and improvements.
- Emergency Preparedness and Response: Strong leadership ensures the development of disaster preparedness plans, early warning systems, and swift responses to health emergencies.
- Capacity Building and Training: Governance supports ongoing capacity building and training for healthcare workers, enabling them to provide high-quality care.
- Ethical Leadership: Ethical leadership models professionalism, integrity, and respect for human rights, setting standards for healthcare providers and inspiring trust in communities.

Conclusion: Enhancing healthcare governance and leadership is a fundamental step toward building resilient communities and robust health systems. By prioritizing transparency, accountability, and inclusivity in decision-making, societies in developing nations can address public health challenges with effectiveness and efficiency. The collective effort to strengthen healthcare governance and leadership contributes to the creation of a responsive, equitable, and resilient healthcare system that empowers communities to navigate health challenges and thrive in the face of adversity [1, 2].

Capacity Building for Healthcare Professionals

Capacity building for healthcare professionals is a cornerstone of building resilient health systems in developing nations. By investing in the continuous development of healthcare workers' knowledge and skills, communities can access higher-quality care, improved clinical practices, and better responses to public health challenges. This section delves into the significance of capacity building for healthcare professionals and outlines strategies for effective implementation [3, 4].

- Continuous Learning Culture: Fostering a culture of continuous learning encourages healthcare professionals to stay updated on the latest medical advancements, techniques, and best practices.

- *Strengthening Primary Healthcare:* Investing in training and empowering primary healthcare workers is essential for providing essential health services at the community level and reducing the burden on tertiary care facilities.
- *Health Workforce Planning:* Strategic health workforce planning can help address workforce shortages and maldistribution, ensuring an adequate and skilled healthcare workforce in all regions.
- *Inclusive Education and Training:* Promoting inclusive education and training opportunities for healthcare professionals from diverse backgrounds can improve cultural competence and equitable healthcare delivery.*Training Programs and Workshops: Organizing regular training programs and workshops on various topics, from clinical skills to public health management, enhances healthcare professionals' competencies.*
- Evidence-Based Practices: Capacity building focuses on equipping healthcare professionals with the skills to use evidence-based practices that lead to better patient outcomes.
- Clinical Guidelines and Protocols: Disseminating and training healthcare professionals in the use of standardized clinical guidelines ensures consistent and high-quality care delivery.
- Specialized Training: Providing specialized training in areas such as emergency response, maternal and child health, and disease management enhances healthcare professionals' ability to address specific health challenges.
- Interdisciplinary Collaboration: Capacity building encourages healthcare professionals to collaborate with colleagues from different disciplines, promoting holistic care and problem-solving.
- Leadership and Management Skills: Healthcare professionals need leadership and management skills to effectively lead teams, allocate resources, and navigate complex healthcare environments.
- Communication and Patient-Centred Care: Training in effective communication and patient-centered care ensures that healthcare professionals prioritize patients' needs and preferences.
- Mental Health and Psychosocial Support Training: Providing training on recognizing and addressing mental health issues equips healthcare professionals to offer holistic care.
- Infection Control and Safety Protocols: Capacity building includes training in infection control, hygiene practices, and safety protocols to protect both patients and healthcare workers.

- Cultural Sensitivity and Equity Training: Training healthcare professionals in cultural sensitivity and equity ensures that care is delivered without bias and respects diverse patient populations.
- Telemedicine and Digital Health Training: As technology becomes integral to healthcare, capacity building includes training in telemedicine platforms and digital health tools.
- Research and Data Analysis Skills: Equipping healthcare professionals with research and data analysis skills promotes evidence-based decision-making and practice improvement.
- *Continuing Professional Development: Encouraging healthcare professionals to pursue continuing education, attend conferences, and engage in lifelong learning enhances their expertise.* Implementing continuous professional development programs ensures that healthcare professionals stay updated with the latest medical advancements, technologies, and best practices.

Conclusion: Capacity building for healthcare professionals is a critical investment in building resilient health systems. By providing ongoing training, skills development, and knowledge enhancement, societies in developing nations can ensure that healthcare professionals are well-equipped to address public health challenges effectively. The collective effort to strengthen healthcare professionals' capacities contributes to the creation of a skilled, adaptable, and empowered healthcare workforce that plays a central role in ensuring the well-being and resilience of communities [3, 4].

Overcoming Challenges in Health System Strengthening

Strengthening health systems is a complex endeavor, particularly in developing nations facing unique challenges. Overcoming these challenges is essential to building resilient communities and ensuring access to quality healthcare. This section discusses the hurdles that may arise during health system strengthening efforts and offers practical solutions for overcoming them [5, 6].

- *Limited Resources:* Insufficient funding and resources can hinder efforts to strengthen health systems, necessitating innovative financing mechanisms and efficient resource allocation.
  - Challenge: Developing nations often face limited financial resources, leading to difficulties in investing adequately in healthcare infrastructure and workforce development.
  - Solution: Prioritize resource allocation based on needs assessment, collaborate with international partners, and explore innovative financing mechanisms such as public-private partnerships.
- Health Workforce Shortages:

- Challenge: Shortages of trained healthcare professionals can impede the delivery of quality care and comprehensive health services.
  - Solution: Implement strategies for recruiting, training, and retaining healthcare workers, including offering incentives, improving working conditions, and promoting professional development.
- Infrastructure and Equipment Gaps:
  - Challenge: Inadequate healthcare facilities and outdated equipment hinder the delivery of timely and effective care.
  - Solution: Invest in infrastructure development, upgrade equipment, and ensure regular maintenance to provide a conducive environment for healthcare services.
- Geographical Barriers:
  - Challenge: Rural and remote areas often have limited access to healthcare due to geographical barriers and inadequate transportation.
  - Solution: Develop mobile health clinics, telemedicine programs, and community health worker networks to extend services to underserved areas.
- *Health Information Systems Challenges:* Strengthening health information systems and data management capacity is critical for evidence-based decision-making and monitoring progress toward health system goals.
  - Challenge: Incomplete or outdated health information systems can hinder data collection, analysis, and informed decision-making.
  - Solution: Invest in robust health information systems, provide training on data management, and ensure interoperability for efficient data sharing.
- Fragmented Healthcare Services:
  - Challenge: Fragmentation in service delivery can result in inefficiencies and gaps in care coordination.
  - Solution: Implement integrated healthcare models, establish referral systems, and promote collaboration among different healthcare providers.
- Cultural and Societal Factors:
  - Challenge: Cultural beliefs, stigmas, and gender disparities can affect healthcare-seeking behaviors and access.
  - Solution: Engage with communities, tailor interventions to cultural norms, and promote gender-sensitive and culturally competent care.
- Weak Governance and Corruption:
  - Challenge: Weak governance and corruption can lead to mismanagement of resources and inefficiencies in healthcare delivery.
  - Solution: Strengthen regulatory frameworks, promote transparency, and engage civil society and watchdog organizations to ensure accountability.
- *Lack of Community Engagement:* Generating political will and aligning diverse stakeholders around health system strengthening goals are essential for sustainable, long-term improvements.

- ○ Challenge: Lack of community involvement in healthcare planning and decision-making can lead to services that do not meet local needs.
- ○ Solution: Engage communities in the design and implementation of health programs, promoting ownership and sustainability.
- Political Instability and Conflict:
  - ○ Challenge: Political instability and conflict can disrupt healthcare services and infrastructure.
  - ○ Solution: Advocate for the protection of healthcare facilities and workers during conflicts and work toward post-conflict recovery plans.
- *Health Inequities and Access Disparities:* Addressing health inequalities and access disparities requires targeted interventions and a focus on reaching vulnerable and marginalized populations.
  - ○ Challenge: Health inequities based on socioeconomic status, gender, and location can lead to unequal access to healthcare.
  - ○ Solution: Implement targeted interventions to address health disparities, prioritize vulnerable populations, and ensure equitable resource allocation.

Conclusion: Overcoming challenges in health system strengthening requires a multi-faceted approach, resilience, and collaborative efforts. By identifying these challenges and implementing tailored solutions, societies in developing nations can build resilient health systems that ensure access to quality care for all. The collective effort to address these obstacles contributes to the creation of healthier communities capable of navigating public health challenges with strength and determination [5, 6].

Case Study 27:*Strengthening Healthcare Governance in a Developing Country.* It explores 'A New Era of Leadership - Strengthening Healthcare Governance.'

Introduction: Effective healthcare governance and leadership are essential for building robust health systems in developing countries. In one developing nation, weak governance had led to fragmented healthcare services and limited access to quality care.

Implementation: To strengthen healthcare governance and leadership, the following initiatives were implemented:

1. Policy Reforms: The government initiated policy reforms to streamline healthcare delivery, improve accountability, and enhance transparency.

2. Health System Integration: Efforts were made to integrate various healthcare services into a unified system, ensuring better coordination and resource allocation.

3. Leadership Training: Healthcare leaders, including administrators and managers, underwent leadership training to enhance their management skills and foster a culture of innovation and improvement.

4. Stakeholder Engagement: Engaging stakeholders, including communities, healthcare professionals, and civil society, in decision-making processes enhanced collaboration and responsiveness.

Results: The efforts to enhance healthcare governance and leadership yielded significant improvements in the health system. Policy reforms led to clearer guidelines and improved resource allocation, resulting in better health service delivery. Health system integration reduced inefficiencies and duplication of services, leading to improved access to comprehensive healthcare. Leadership training improved the management capabilities of healthcare leaders, resulting in better decision-making and implementation of innovative solutions. Stakeholder engagement fostered a sense of ownership and empowerment, leading to greater community involvement in healthcare initiatives. Overall, the strengthened healthcare governance and leadership transformed the health system, making it more efficient, responsive, and accountable.

Case Study 28:*Capacity Building for Healthcare Professionals in Rural Settings.* It looks at 'Empowering Rural Healthcare - Capacity Building for Healthcare Professionals.'

Introduction: Rural healthcare settings in developing nations often face a shortage of skilled healthcare professionals, hindering the delivery of quality care. In one remote rural area, capacity-building initiatives were undertaken to address this challenge.

Implementation: To enhance the capacity of healthcare professionals in the rural area, the following measures were taken:

1. Continuous Medical Education: Regular training programs and workshops were conducted to update healthcare professionals' medical knowledge and skills.

2. Specialized Training: Healthcare professionals received specialized training in managing prevalent health issues specific to the rural context, such as infectious diseases and maternal and child health.

3. Telemedicine Support: Telemedicine platforms were introduced to provide remote consultations and guidance from specialists, enabling healthcare professionals to manage complex cases effectively.

4. Incentives and Support: Incentives, such as scholarships and career advancement opportunities, were provided to encourage healthcare professionals to work in rural areas.

Results: The capacity-building initiatives led to a noticeable improvement in healthcare services in the rural area. Continuous medical education empowered healthcare professionals with updated knowledge and best practices, improving the quality of care they delivered. Specialized training enhanced the management of prevalent health issues, leading to better health outcomes for the rural population. Telemedicine support improved access to expert advice and consultation, particularly for complex cases. The incentives and support provided motivated healthcare professionals to stay and serve in rural areas, addressing the shortage of skilled workforce. As a result, the rural healthcare setting demonstrated increased capacity, competence, and effectiveness in delivering healthcare services to the community.

Conclusion: These case studies exemplify the importance of enhancing healthcare governance and leadership, capacity building for healthcare professionals, and overcoming challenges in health system strengthening. By focusing on effective governance, leadership training, and stakeholder engagement, health systems can become more responsive, accountable, and integrated. Capacity-building initiatives, combined with telemedicine support and incentives, can improve the skill set and retention of healthcare professionals, particularly in underserved areas. Strengthening health systems and governance is integral to achieving equitable and efficient healthcare services, paving the way for improved health outcomes in developing nations.

CONCLUSION

Strengthening health systems and governance is a complex but essential undertaking for improving health outcomes and achieving universal health coverage. By prioritizing effective governance structures, investing in healthcare capacity building, and addressing challenges through innovative solutions, societies can build resilient health systems capable of responding to public health challenges and promoting the well-being of all individuals.

REFERENCES

[1]   World Health Organization. Health System Governance: Effective Health System Governance for Universal Health Coverage UHC. World Health Organization, 2021. Available from: https://www.who.int/health-topics/health-systems-governance#tab=tab_1

[2]   Kruk ME, Gage AD, Joseph NT, Danaei G, García-Saisó S, Salomon JA. Mortality due to low-quality health systems in the universal health coverage era: a systematic analysis of amenable deaths in 137 countries. Lancet 2018; 392(10160): 2203-12.
[http://dx.doi.org/10.1016/S0140-6736(18)31668-4] [PMID: 30195398]

[3]   World Health Organization. Transformative scale-up of health professional education: an effort to increase the numbers of health professionals and to strengthen their impact on population health. World Health Organization, 2011. Available from: https://apps.who.int/iris/handle/10665/70573

[4]   Frenk J, Chen L, Bhutta ZA, *et al.* Health professionals for a new century: transforming education to strengthen health systems in an interdependent world. Lancet 2010; 376(9756): 1923-58.
[http://dx.doi.org/10.1016/S0140-6736(10)61854-5] [PMID: 21112623]

[5]   World Health Organization. Strengthening Health Systems to Improve Health Outcomes: WHO's Framework for Action. World Health Organization, 2007. Available from: https://apps.who.int/iris/bitstream/handle/10665/43918/9789241596077_eng.pdf

[6]   Agyepong IA, Sewankambo N, Binagwaho A, *et al.* The path to longer and healthier lives for all Africans by 2030: the Lancet Commission on the future of health in sub-Saharan Africa. Lancet 2017; 390(10114): 2803-59.
[http://dx.doi.org/10.1016/S0140-6736(17)31509-X] [PMID: 28917958]

CHAPTER 16

Sustainable Development and Resilient Health Futures

Abstract: Sustainable development and resilient health systems are crucial for building a healthier and more equitable future for developing nations. This chapter explores the integration of public health into sustainable development goals, the importance of fostering long-term resilience in communities, and strategies for shaping a healthier future. By aligning public health efforts with sustainable development objectives, promoting community resilience, and embracing forward-thinking approaches, developing nations can overcome health challenges and create a brighter and more sustainable future for their populations.

Keywords: Community resilience, Developing nations, Integration, Public health, Resilient health systems, Sustainable development.

INTRODUCTION

Aligning public health efforts with the United Nations Sustainable Development Goals (SDGs) is essential for building resilient communities and fostering sustainable development. Recognizing the interconnectedness of health with poverty reduction, education, gender equality, and environmental protection is key. Strategies include data-driven decision-making, cross-sectoral collaboration, and empowering vulnerable populations. By integrating public health into the broader SDG framework, societies can promote holistic development that addresses the well-being of individuals, communities, and the planet.

Building long-term resilience in communities is critical for their ability to withstand shocks and sustain positive health outcomes. Strategies for fostering resilience include investing in local capacity, disaster risk reduction, health education, and economic empowerment. By empowering communities to drive their development and promoting inclusivity and sustainability, societies can build resilient communities capable of overcoming adversity and contributing to broader sustainable development goals.

Shaping a healthier future for developing nations requires a collective commitment to public health and sustainable development principles. Strategies include strengthening health systems, promoting environmental and climate health, and investing in human capital. By prioritizing equity, innovation, and multi-sectoral collaboration, societies can create a future where health is central to development, resilience is embedded in communities, and individuals are empowered to thrive.

Integrating Public Health into Sustainable Development Goals

The United Nations Sustainable Development Goals (SDGs) provide a comprehensive framework for addressing global challenges, including public health issues, poverty, inequality, environmental degradation, and more. Integrating public health into the SDGs is a crucial step toward building resilient communities and fostering sustainable development in developing nations. This section delves into the significance of aligning public health efforts with the SDGs and outlines strategies for integration [1, 2].

- *The 2030 Agenda for Sustainable Development:* The United Nations' 2030 Agenda sets forth 17 Sustainable Development Goals (SDGs) with 169 targets, aiming to address global challenges, including poverty, hunger, health, education, gender equality, and climate change.
- *Goal 3 - Good Health and Well-being:* SDG 3 specifically focuses on ensuring healthy lives and promoting well-being for all ages. It calls for various targets, such as reducing maternal and child mortality, combating communicable and non-communicable diseases, and achieving universal health coverage.
- The Interconnectedness of Goals: Recognize that public health is intrinsically linked to various SDGs, including Goal 3 (Good Health and Well-being), Goal 1 (No Poverty), Goal 2 (Zero Hunger), Goal 6 (Clean Water and Sanitation), Goal 4 (Quality Education), and others.
- Holistic Approach to Health: Understand that health outcomes are influenced by social, economic, and environmental factors, necessitating a comprehensive approach that addresses the root causes of health disparities.
- Health as a Catalyst for Development: Realize that improving health outcomes contributes to poverty reduction, economic growth, and overall human development, creating a positive cycle of progress.
- Data-Driven Decision-Making: Leverage data to identify health priorities within the context of sustainable development, guiding resource allocation and intervention strategies.
- Cross-Sectoral Collaboration: Promote collaboration between health sectors and other relevant sectors, such as education, water and sanitation, agriculture, and environmental protection, to achieve integrated solutions. Integrating public health into the broader sustainable development agenda requires collaboration across various sectors, including health, education, environment, and finance, to

address the underlying social determinants of health.

- *Addressing Health Inequalities:* To achieve sustainable health outcomes, it is crucial to address health inequalities and disparities, both within and between countries, to ensure that no one is left behind in accessing essential health services.
- Policy Coherence: Ensure that health policies are aligned with broader development policies, promoting synergy and minimizing conflicting priorities.
- Community Participation: Engage communities in the SDG process to ensure that health interventions and development initiatives meet local needs and priorities.
- Empowering Vulnerable Populations: Prioritize the health and well-being of marginalized and vulnerable populations, as their inclusion is central to achieving the SDGs.
- Environmental Health Nexus: Recognize the impact of environmental factors on public health and the environment's role in achieving health and well-being goals.
- Innovative Financing Mechanisms: Explore innovative funding approaches that support both health and sustainable development objectives, such as impact investments and public-private partnerships.
- Health System Strengthening: View health system strengthening as a critical enabler of achieving multiple SDGs, particularly Goal 3, by improving access to quality healthcare.
- Behavioral Change and Education: Promote health education and behavior change campaigns that align with SDGs, encouraging individuals to adopt sustainable and healthy lifestyles.
- Advocacy and Awareness: Advocate for the integration of health considerations into SDG-related policies and raise awareness about the interconnected nature of health and development.
- Monitoring and Reporting: Track progress on health-related indicators within the SDG framework, demonstrating the impact of health initiatives on sustainable development outcomes.

Conclusion: Integrating public health into the Sustainable Development Goals represents a powerful approach to building resilient communities and promoting sustainable development in developing nations. By recognizing the intricate connections between health and broader development objectives, societies can foster a more equitable, prosperous, and resilient future for all. The collective effort to align public health initiatives with the SDGs contributes to a holistic approach to development that addresses the well-being of individuals, communities, and the planet [1, 2].

Fostering Long-Term Resilience in Communities

Building long-term resilience in communities is essential for their ability to navigate challenges, adapt to changes, and sustain positive health outcomes over time. This section delves into the importance of fostering enduring resilience within communities and outlines strategies for promoting sustainable development that prioritizes health and well-being [3, 4].

- *Community Resilience as a Concept:* Community resilience refers to a community's ability to bounce back and recover from shocks and stresses, including health emergencies and disasters.
- *Building Social Capital:* Social cohesion, community engagement, and strong social networks contribute to building social capital, which enhances communities' ability to cope with challenges collectively. Cultivate strong social networks within communities that provide support, information sharing, and mutual assistance during times of adversity.
- *Investing in Local Capacity:* Strengthening local capacities, including community organizations, healthcare providers, and disaster response teams, enhances preparedness and response capabilities.
- *Disaster Risk Reduction:* Incorporating disaster risk reduction measures into community planning and development helps mitigate the impact of disasters on public health.
- Community-Led Approaches: Empower communities to drive their own development and health initiatives, ensuring that interventions align with their needs, strengths, and cultural context.
- Health Education and Empowerment: Provide ongoing health education that empowers individuals to make informed decisions about their health and encourages healthy behaviors and lifestyles.
- Capacity Building and Skill Development: Equip community members with essential skills, such as first aid, basic healthcare knowledge, and disaster preparedness, enabling them to respond effectively to emergencies.
- Diversified Livelihoods: Promote economic diversification and skill development to enhance communities' ability to secure income and resources even in the face of economic fluctuations.
- Infrastructure and Environmental Resilience: Invest in resilient infrastructure, such as disaster-resistant housing and water supply systems, to minimize vulnerability to environmental shocks.
- Local Resource Management: Encourage sustainable management of local resources, such as water, land, and forests, to support long-term community well-being.
- Gender Equality and Social Inclusion: Ensure that resilience-building efforts prioritize gender equality and include marginalized and vulnerable populations

to create a more inclusive and equitable community.

- Early Warning Systems: Establish community-based early warning systems for disease outbreaks, natural disasters, and other emergencies to enable swift response and evacuation.
- Adaptive Planning and Flexibility: Develop adaptive planning processes that allow communities to adjust strategies in response to changing circumstances and emerging challenges.
- Knowledge Sharing and Learning: Foster a culture of continuous learning, where communities share knowledge and experiences to improve their collective resilience strategies.
- Disaster Preparedness Drills: Conduct regular disaster preparedness drills that involve the entire community, ensuring that everyone knows their role during emergencies.
- Partnerships and Collaboration: Forge partnerships with local governments, NGOs, academic institutions, and other stakeholders to pool resources, expertise, and support.
- Long-Term Sustainability: Ensure that resilience-building initiatives are sustainable over time, incorporating mechanisms for ongoing funding, maintenance, and community engagement.

Conclusion: Fostering long-term resilience within communities is a multifaceted endeavor that requires collaboration, empowerment, and a commitment to sustainable development. By prioritizing health, education, economic empowerment, and community engagement, societies in developing nations can build communities that not only withstand health challenges but also thrive and contribute to broader sustainable development goals. The collective effort to foster enduring resilience leads to communities that are equipped to overcome adversity and create a healthier, more prosperous, and resilient future for generations to come [3, 4].

Shaping a Healthier Future for Developing Nations

As developing nations navigate the intricate landscape of public health challenges and sustainable development, the opportunity to shape a healthier future for their populations becomes paramount. This section delves into the significance of aligning public health with sustainable development and outlines strategies for creating a brighter and more resilient future for developing nations [5, 6].

- *Strengthening Health Systems:* Investing in robust health systems is essential for achieving sustainable health outcomes. This includes enhancing healthcare infrastructure, ensuring a skilled health workforce, and improving health information systems.

- *Primary Healthcare as a Foundation:* Strong primary healthcare serves as the foundation for delivering essential health services and promoting preventive care at the community level.
- *Addressing Environmental and Climate Health:* Environmental and climate health considerations are critical in shaping a healthier future, as they affect air and water quality, food security, and disease transmission.
- *Promoting Health Education and Literacy:* Health education and literacy initiatives empower individuals and communities to make informed decisions about their health, leading to better health-seeking behaviors. Prioritize education on health, hygiene, and sustainable practices to empower individuals to make informed decisions about their well-being.
- Vision of Holistic Well-being: Envision a future where health is not just the absence of disease but a state of complete physical, mental, and social well-being, driving development efforts.
- Health as a Pillar of Development: Recognize health as a fundamental building block of sustainable development, influencing economic growth, education, and social equity.
- Investment in Human Capital: View health as an investment in human capital, enabling individuals to reach their full potential and contribute to the development of their communities and nations.
- Equity and Inclusivity: Commit to achieving health equity, ensuring that all individuals, regardless of their background or circumstances, have equal access to quality healthcare and opportunities.
- Resilience as a Core Value: Embed resilience-building into the fabric of society, empowering communities to proactively adapt to challenges and minimize their impact.
- Innovation and Technology: Harness the power of innovation and technology to enhance healthcare delivery, data collection, and resource management for better health outcomes.
- Multi-Sectoral Collaboration: Promote collaboration across sectors, breaking down silos to address complex health challenges through integrated and holistic approaches.
- Community Engagement: Foster active community participation in health and development initiatives, ensuring that solutions are tailored to local needs and context.
- Environmental Stewardship: Promote environmental conservation and sustainable resource management, recognizing the interdependence between a healthy environment and public health.
- Data-Driven Decision-Making: Base policy and planning decisions on accurate and timely health data, enabling evidence-based interventions and resource allocation.

- Policy Coherence and Governance: Ensure alignment between health policies and broader development goals, supported by effective governance and transparent decision-making.
- Empowering Women and Girls: Recognize the critical role of gender equality in achieving better health outcomes and promoting women's access to education, healthcare, and decision-making.
- Continuous Adaptation: Adopt a mindset of continuous adaptation and learning, allowing nations to respond effectively to emerging health challenges and changing circumstances.

Conclusion: Shaping a healthier future for developing nations requires a collective commitment to the intertwined goals of public health and sustainable development. By prioritizing health as a foundational element of progress and resilience, societies can foster well-being, equity, and prosperity for generations to come. The efforts to align public health initiatives with sustainable development principles contribute to a future where communities are empowered, resilient, and poised to overcome challenges while building a healthier and more vibrant society [5, 6].

Case Study 29: *Integrating Public Health into Sustainable Development Goals.* It looks at 'A Holistic Approach - Integrating Public Health and Sustainable Development.'

Introduction: Sustainable development is closely linked to public health, as health outcomes significantly impact a nation's progress and prosperity. In one developing nation, a comprehensive approach was adopted to integrate public health into sustainable development goals.

Implementation: To integrate public health into sustainable development goals, the following strategies were implemented:

1. Intersectoral Collaboration: Different government departments, including health, education, environment, and agriculture, collaborated to address health challenges holistically.

2. Health Impact Assessments: Health impact assessments were conducted for policies and projects to identify potential health risks and opportunities for promoting well-being.

3. Health-Inclusive Development Plans: Sustainable development plans were formulated to incorporate health indicators and goals, ensuring health was a priority in all development initiatives.

4. Empowering Local Communities: Local communities were actively involved in decision-making processes, ensuring their health needs and perspectives were considered in development projects.

Results: The integration of public health into sustainable development goals yielded positive outcomes. Intersectoral collaboration led to more comprehensive and effective policies and programs, addressing health determinants beyond the healthcare sector. Health impact assessments improved the overall health impact of development projects, preventing potential negative consequences on health. Health-inclusive development plans resulted in a stronger focus on public health, leading to improved health indicators and well-being in the population. Empowering local communities enhanced community resilience and ownership, fostering sustainability and long-term health benefits. The integration of public health and sustainable development goals created a mutually reinforcing relationship, laying the foundation for a healthier and more resilient future for the nation.

Case Study 30: *Fostering Long-Term Resilience in a Vulnerable Community.* It explores 'Rising Above Adversities - Fostering Resilience in a Vulnerable Community.'

Introduction: Vulnerable communities in developing nations face multiple challenges, including health disparities, environmental hazards, and limited resources. In one such vulnerable community, a resilience-building initiative was undertaken to address these complex challenges.

Implementation: To foster long-term resilience in the vulnerable community, the following initiatives were implemented:

1. Community-Based Planning: A participatory approach was adopted, engaging community members in identifying their unique challenges and designing locally relevant resilience strategies.

2. Diversified Livelihoods: Efforts were made to diversify livelihood opportunities, reducing dependence on single income sources and building economic resilience.

3. Disaster Preparedness and Response: The community received training in disaster preparedness and response, equipping them to cope with environmental hazards and emergencies effectively.

4. Environmental Sustainability: Environmental conservation and sustainable resource management were promoted, ensuring long-term ecological resilience.

Results: The resilience-building initiative had a transformative impact on the vulnerable community. Community-based planning led to tailored interventions that addressed the community's specific needs and vulnerabilities. Diversified livelihoods provided economic stability, reducing vulnerability to shocks and improving the community's adaptive capacity. Disaster preparedness and response training enhanced the community's ability to withstand and recover from disasters, minimizing health risks and losses. Emphasizing environmental sustainability ensured the community's long-term resilience and safeguarded natural resources essential for health and well-being. As a result, the vulnerable community demonstrated improved resilience, health outcomes, and prospects for a sustainable and healthier future.

Conclusion: These case studies illustrate the significance of integrating public health into sustainable development goals, fostering long-term resilience in communities, and shaping a healthier future for developing nations. By adopting intersectoral collaboration, health impact assessments, and health-inclusive development plans, public health can be seamlessly integrated into sustainable development initiatives, promoting equitable and inclusive growth. Fostering long-term resilience in vulnerable communities requires empowering local stakeholders, diversifying livelihoods, and emphasizing environmental sustainability. These strategies can collectively contribute to building more resilient, healthier, and sustainable futures for developing nations, ensuring the well-being and prosperity of present and future generations.

CONCLUSION

Integrating public health into sustainable development goals, fostering long-term resilience in communities, and shaping a healthier future are interconnected efforts essential for building robust and equitable health systems in developing nations. By aligning public health initiatives with sustainable development objectives, promoting community resilience, and embracing forward-thinking approaches, societies can overcome health challenges and create a brighter and more sustainable future for their populations.

REFERENCES

[1]   United Nations. Transforming Our World: The 2030 Agenda for Sustainable Development. United Nations, 2015. Available from: https://sdgs.un.org/2030agenda

[2]   World Health Assembly, 69. Health in the 2030 Agenda for Sustainable Development. World Health Organization, 2016. Available from: https://apps.who.int/iris/handle/10665/252791

[3]   Norris FH, Stevens SP, Pfefferbaum B, Wyche KF, Pfefferbaum RL. Community resilience as a metaphor, theory, set of capacities, and strategy for disaster readiness. Am J Community Psychol 2008; 41(1-2): 127-50.
[http://dx.doi.org/10.1007/s10464-007-9156-6] [PMID: 18157631]

[4]   Patel, S. S., Rogers, M. B., Amlôt, R., & Rubin, G. J. What Do We Mean by 'Community Resilience'? A Systematic Literature Review of How It Is Defined in the Literature. PLoS currents, 2017; 9.

[5]   World Health Organization. Working for a brighter, healthier future: how WHO improves health and promotes well-being for the world's adolescents. Geneva: World Health Organization; 2021. Licence: CC BY-NC-SA 3.0 IGO.

[6]   Global Burden of Disease Collaborative Network. Global Burden of Disease Study 2019 (GBD 2019) Results. Institute for Health Metrics and Evaluation (IHME), 2019. Available from: https://www.healthdata.org/research-analysis/gbd

CHAPTER 17

Overcoming Key Public Health Challenges

Abstract: This chapter provides a comprehensive examination of critical public health challenges in developing nations, emphasising the essential role of resilient communities in addressing these issues. Key challenges discussed include weak routine immunisation, poor leadership and governance, poor coordination of disease outbreak and response, and non-performing primary healthcare centres. Resilient communities demonstrate proactive engagement through advocacy, collaboration, and innovation, showcasing their transformative potential in creating healthier and more resilient societies.

Keywords: Advocacy, Collaboration, Disease outbreak, Developing nations, Governance, Empowerment, Leadership, Public health challenges, Primary healthcare centers, Resilient communities, Routine immunization.

INTRODUCTION

In the ever-evolving landscape of global health, addressing public health challenges in developing nations remains a multifaceted endeavour, shaped by diverse factors that define the health and well-being of populations. Nowhere are these challenges more pronounced and compelling than in developing nations, where a complex and interconnected web of issues converges, giving rise to unique health disparities and formidable obstacles. This section sets the stage for an in-depth exploration of the critical issues surrounding weak routine immunisation, poor leadership and governance in health, poor coordination of disease outbreaks and response, and non-performing primary healthcare facilities.

The previous chapters of this book emphasise the pivotal role that resilient communities play in addressing these challenges. Resilient communities are not passive bystanders but active participants in shaping their health destinies. They catalyse change, inspiring hope and progress despite seemingly insurmountable challenges. Their success stories serve as beacons of light, illuminating the transformative potential of community-driven initiatives and local-level action.

Weak Routine Immunization: A Looming Threat

Routine immunisation is not merely a public health strategy; it is a shield that protects communities from the devastating impact of vaccine-preventable diseases. It is the cornerstone of global health efforts, ensuring that children and adults are shielded from various ailments, from measles and polio to diphtheria and influenza. However, in many developing nations, the threat of weak routine immunisation casts a long shadow, and its consequences are both immediate and long-lasting [1, 2].

The Threat of Weakened Immunization Programs

One of the most significant challenges facing developing nations is the weakening of routine immunisation programs. Several factors contribute to this perilous scenario, including limited resources, inadequate infrastructure, logistical challenges, and a lack of awareness among communities. As a result, many children and adults are left susceptible to vaccine-preventable diseases that could have been averted through timely and comprehensive immunisation.

Consequences for Public Health

The consequences of weak routine immunisation programs are profound and far-reaching. At the individual level, the lack of immunisation leaves children vulnerable to debilitating and life-threatening diseases. These diseases cause suffering and can disrupt education, impede economic well-being, and exacerbate existing social disparities.

At the community level, weak immunisation programs compromise herd immunity, which is essential for preventing the spread of diseases. Communities with low vaccination rates are more susceptible to outbreaks, and this vulnerability can extend to neighbouring areas. Disease outbreaks, such as measles or whooping cough, have the potential to strain already overburdened healthcare systems in developing nations.

Resilient Communities' Response

However, within this looming threat lies an opportunity for resilient communities to take the initiative. Resilient communities recognise the importance of routine immunisation, and they actively engage in raising awareness, advocating for access to vaccines, and ensuring that healthcare systems prioritise immunisation services. They harness their local knowledge, social networks, and community-driven initiatives to overcome barriers that weaken immunisation programs.

Resilient communities protect their members by actively seeking immunisation and serving as role models for others. By demonstrating the benefits of routine immunisation, they can inspire neighbouring communities to follow suit, creating a ripple effect that strengthens immunisation efforts on a broader scale.

Innovative Solutions

In the face of the looming threat of weak routine immunisation, communities are finding innovative solutions. Mobile vaccination clinics, community health workers, and local education campaigns are some of the approaches that have successfully increased immunisation rates. These solutions reflect the adaptability and resourcefulness of resilient communities when faced with challenges.

Global Collaboration and Support

Addressing weak routine immunisation is not the sole responsibility of communities. It requires a coordinated effort involving governments, international organisations, non-governmental entities, and community leaders. Resilient communities actively seek partnerships and support to bolster their immunisation efforts, emphasising the need for access to vaccines and resources.

In conclusion, the looming threat of weak routine immunisation is a critical challenge in developing nations, and its consequences can be severe. However, it is a challenge that resilient communities are addressing head-on. By emphasising the importance of routine immunisation, advocating for its accessibility, and implementing innovative strategies, these communities serve as beacons of hope in the fight against vaccine-preventable diseases. They remind us that, even in the face of this looming threat, communities can unite, overcome obstacles, and protect the health of their members.

Poor Leadership and Governance: Barriers to Progress

Effective leadership and governance are fundamental pillars of successful public health systems. They provide the strategic direction, resource allocation, and oversight required to address complex health challenges. However, in many developing nations, poor leadership and governance pose significant barriers to progress, hindering the delivery of essential healthcare services and eroding public trust in health systems [3, 4].

The Impact of Ineffective Leadership and Governance

- *Mismanagement:* Weak or ineffective leadership can result in mismanagement of resources and priorities. This often leads to inefficiencies in healthcare delivery, misallocation of funds, and a lack of accountability in public health initiatives.

- *Resource Allocation Issues:* Sound governance is critical for the equitable allocation of resources. Ineffective governance can result in disparities in resource distribution, favouring urban areas while neglecting rural and underserved communities. This exacerbates healthcare inequalities and prevents equitable access to services.
- *Lack of Strategic Planning:* Effective leadership and governance are responsible for setting strategic goals and planning for the long-term improvement of healthcare systems. In the absence of strategic planning, healthcare systems struggle to adapt to changing circumstances, and their capacity to respond to crises is compromised.
- *Diminished Accountability:* Weak governance often leads to a lack of accountability, where individuals responsible for healthcare management escape consequences for mismanagement, corruption, or malpractice. This erodes public trust in health systems and impedes progress.

Strategies for Improving Leadership and Governance

Addressing the issue of poor leadership and governance is crucial for making progress in public health in developing nations. Resilient communities, in collaboration with various stakeholders, can play an instrumental role in driving change and improving leadership and governance:

- *Advocacy and Transparency:* Resilient communities can advocate for transparent and accountable governance structures. They can push for transparency in budget allocations and hold leaders accountable for their actions. Transparency is a cornerstone of effective governance.
- *Capacity Building:* Building leadership and governance capacity is essential. Resilient communities can actively engage in training programs for future leaders, helping to create a pool of individuals who are knowledgeable and committed to improving public health systems.
- *Community Involvement:* Resilient communities can actively participate in community health committees and health planning processes. This empowers them to have a say in resource allocation and healthcare service priorities, ensuring that local needs are addressed.
- *Collaboration with External Partners:* Resilient communities can partner with non-governmental organisations, international agencies, and public health professionals to create partnerships that foster good governance practices. These external partners can provide technical expertise and resources to strengthen governance structures.

Challenges and the Path Forward

The path to improving leadership and governance is not without its challenges. Entrenched interests, political factors, and resistance to change can all pose obstacles. However, the tenacity and determination of resilient communities are powerful drivers of change.

Through advocacy, transparency, community involvement, and collaboration with external partners, resilient communities can actively contribute to transforming leadership and governance in public health. They can serve as catalysts for accountability, demand excellence in healthcare management, and ultimately create more effective and responsive public health systems.

In conclusion, poor leadership and governance are formidable barriers to progress in public health in developing nations. However, resilient communities are not passive bystanders but active participants in driving change. By advocating for transparency, building capacity, engaging in community planning, and collaborating with external partners, they can help pave the way for more effective and equitable leadership and governance in public health. Their resilience and determination provide hope for the future of public health systems in these nations.

Poor Coordination of Disease Outbreak and Response

Effective coordination in the face of disease outbreaks is paramount to mitigate their impact and save lives. Poor coordination of disease outbreaks and response poses a significant challenge in many developing nations, amplifying the threat of infectious diseases and hampering the ability to respond swiftly and effectively. In this section, we delve into the complexities of this issue, its consequences, and the role of resilient communities in improving coordination during health crises [5 - 7].

The Challenge of Coordinating Disease Outbreak Response

- *Logistical Complexities:* Coordinating the response to a disease outbreak, especially in resource-limited settings, is fraught with logistical challenges. These include ensuring the timely delivery of medical supplies, deploying healthcare personnel, and managing quarantine and isolation facilities.
- *Fragmented Healthcare Systems:* Many developing nations grapple with fragmented healthcare systems, hindering the seamless flow of information and resources during an outbreak. Fragmentation can lead to a lack of consistency in response strategies.

- *Communication Barriers:* Effective communication is pivotal in outbreak response, but language barriers, inadequate communication infrastructure, and a lack of standardised communication protocols can hinder information sharing.
- *Resource Constraints:* Limited resources, both human and financial, can constrain the ability to respond comprehensively to an outbreak. Overstretched healthcare facilities may struggle to provide care, while the shortage of trained personnel can impede response efforts.

Consequences of Poor Coordination

- *Delayed Response:* A lack of coordination often results in delayed responses to outbreaks, allowing diseases to spread further. Delays can increase morbidity and mortality rates, especially in cases of highly contagious diseases.
- *Inefficient Resource Allocation:* Resources may be misallocated or duplicated, wasting precious time and assets. This inefficiency can weaken the overall response and prolong the duration of an outbreak.
- *Community Distrust:* Poor coordination can erode public trust in healthcare systems, making communities less likely to comply with containment measures. This distrust can further exacerbate the outbreak.

Resilient Communities as Agents of Improved Coordination

Resilient communities recognise the importance of coordination in outbreak response, and they actively contribute to its enhancement in several ways:

- *Local Response Teams:* Resilient communities can establish local response teams comprised of individuals with training in outbreak management. These teams can help bridge the gap between healthcare facilities and the community.
- *Community Education:* By educating their members about outbreak response protocols and preventive measures, resilient communities ensure that individuals are informed and can act proactively.
- *Support for Healthcare Workers:* Resilient communities can support healthcare workers by assisting in contact tracing, providing psychosocial support to affected individuals, and helping with resource mobilisation.
- *Community Surveillance:* Community members can actively participate in surveillance efforts by reporting symptoms and cases promptly, contributing to early detection and containment.

Collaboration and Partnerships

To address the challenge of poor coordination, collaboration and partnerships are essential. Resilient communities can collaborate with healthcare professionals, local authorities, and non-governmental organisations to establish effective response systems. These partnerships can foster better information sharing, resource allocation, and the timely implementation of control measures.

In conclusion, poor coordination of disease outbreaks and response is a significant challenge in developing nations, with far-reaching consequences. Resilient communities are crucial in improving coordination during health crises by establishing response teams, educating their members, and actively participating in surveillance efforts. Collaborative efforts with healthcare professionals and external partners can further strengthen response systems, enhancing the resilience of communities and the effectiveness of outbreak response efforts.

Non-Performing Primary Healthcare Centers: Bridging the Gap

Primary healthcare centres are the backbone of any healthcare system, providing essential and accessible medical services to communities. However, in many developing nations, the non-performance of primary healthcare centres presents a formidable challenge, limiting access to vital healthcare services. In this section, we delve into the issues surrounding absent or non-performing primary healthcare centres, their impact on public health, and the crucial role of resilient communities in bridging this gap [8 - 10].

The Challenge of Non-Performing Primary Healthcare Centers

• *Lack of Infrastructure:* In some regions, primary healthcare centres are nonexistent due to a lack of infrastructure. This absence leaves communities without a local source of basic medical care, forcing them to travel long distances to seek treatment.
• *Inadequate Staffing:* Even when primary healthcare centres exist, they may suffer from inadequate staffing, with a shortage of trained healthcare professionals. This can lead to long wait times and suboptimal care.
• *Resource Constraints:* Primary healthcare centres often lack the necessary resources, such as medical supplies and equipment, to provide quality care. Resource constraints can compromise the effectiveness of these centres.
• *Geographic Disparities:* In many cases, primary healthcare centres are concentrated in urban areas, leaving rural and remote communities with limited or no access to healthcare services.

Consequences of Non-Performing Primary Healthcare Centers

• *Limited Access to Care:* The non-performance of primary healthcare centres limits access to basic healthcare services, including preventive care, early disease diagnosis, and treatment of common illnesses.

- *Increased Health Disparities:* Communities without access to primary healthcare centres often face higher morbidity and mortality rates, leading to increased health disparities and inequities.
- *Economic Burden:* Individuals and families must bear the economic burden of travelling long distances to access healthcare services, including transportation costs and lost wages.

Resilient Communities as Agents of Change

Resilient communities recognise that access to healthcare is a fundamental right, and they actively work to bridge the gap created by absent or non-performing primary healthcare centres:

- *Community-Managed Healthcare:* Resilient communities can establish community-managed healthcare initiatives, which include locally trained healthcare workers who can provide basic care services.
- *Resource Mobilisation*: Communities can mobilise financial and material resources to support the functioning of primary healthcare centres. This includes fundraising efforts and advocacy for government investment in healthcare infrastructure.
- *Advocacy for Access*: Resilient communities are vocal advocates for access to healthcare services. They actively engage with local authorities and healthcare policymakers to highlight the importance of primary healthcare centres and their role in improving community health.
- *Local Health Education*: Resilient communities prioritise health education programs, helping community members understand the importance of preventive care and timely access to healthcare services.

Collaboration and Partnerships

To address the challenge of non-performing primary healthcare centres, collaboration with healthcare professionals, local authorities, and non-governmental organisations is crucial. These partnerships can lead to the establishment of community healthcare centres, the allocation of resources, and the provision of training for community health workers.

In conclusion, the non-performance of primary healthcare centres poses a significant challenge in developing nations, limiting access to essential healthcare services. Resilient communities actively engage in efforts to bridge this gap by establishing community-managed healthcare initiatives, advocating for access, and mobilising resources. Collaborative efforts with healthcare professionals and external partners can further strengthen the role of primary healthcare centres and improve community health outcomes, ultimately contributing to the resilience and well-being of communities.

Resilient Communities as Agents of Change

Resilient communities are powerful catalysts for positive change in the context of public health in developing nations. They are not passive recipients of aid or solutions but active participants who take ownership of their health and well-being. This section explores the pivotal role that resilient communities play as agents of change in improving public health, emphasising their characteristics, actions, and impact [11 - 13].

Characteristics of Resilient Communities

- *Empowerment:* Resilient communities are empowered communities. They recognise their agency in addressing health challenges and are actively involved in decision-making. Empowerment leads to a sense of ownership and responsibility for community health.
- *Adaptability:* Resilient communities exhibit adaptability in the face of adversity. They quickly respond to changing circumstances and seek innovative solutions to health challenges, even with limited resources.
- *Community Cohesion:* Strong social bonds and community cohesion are hallmarks of resilient communities. These bonds promote collective action, unity, and support, enabling communities to tackle health challenges as a team.
- *Resourcefulness:* Resilient communities are resourceful and creative. They make the most of their available resources, whether through innovative healthcare delivery models, local knowledge, or community-driven initiatives.
- *Advocacy:* Resilient communities are vocal advocates for their health needs. They engage with local authorities, healthcare professionals, and policymakers to ensure their concerns are heard and addressed.

Actions of Resilient Communities

- *Community Health Initiatives:* Resilient communities initiate and manage their health programs, including awareness campaigns, disease prevention efforts, and local healthcare services. They take the lead in shaping health interventions that are tailored to their specific needs and context.
- *Capacity Building:* Resilient communities actively engage in capacity-building efforts, including training community health workers and educating community members. They aim to build a skilled and informed local workforce capable of addressing health challenges.
- *Collaboration and Partnerships:* Resilient communities foster partnerships with various stakeholders, including healthcare professionals, non-governmental

organisations, and government agencies. These collaborations enhance their access to resources and technical expertise.

- *Advocacy and Policy Influence:* Resilient communities advocate for health policy changes, prioritising their well-being. They influence local, regional, and national decisions, ensuring their voices are heard in shaping public health policies.

Impact of Resilient Communities

- *Improved Health Outcomes:* Resilient communities actively contribute to improved health outcomes by proactively addressing health challenges, implementing preventive measures, and ensuring timely access to healthcare services.
- *Health Equity:* Resilient communities are champions of health equity. Their actions prioritise marginalised and vulnerable populations, ensuring no one is left behind in health interventions.
- *Community Well-Being:* Resilient communities enhance overall community well-being, focusing not only on physical health but also on the social, economic, and environmental determinants of health.
- *Inspiration and Replication:* Resilient communities serve as sources of inspiration for neighbouring communities. Their successful initiatives and approaches often inspire others to replicate their efforts, creating a ripple effect of positive change.

In conclusion, resilient communities are essential agents of change in the field of public health in developing nations. Their characteristics, actions, and impact demonstrate the transformative potential of local-level action and community-driven initiatives. Resilient communities remind us that, despite formidable health challenges, the collective power of communities can lead to improved health outcomes, health equity, and the creation of healthier and more resilient societies.

Conclusion: "Resilient Communities: Navigating Public Health Challenges in Developing Nations" has taken us on a journey through the intricate tapestry of public health challenges in the context of resource-constrained settings. In these developing nations, where communities face daunting health disparities and obstacles, the significance of resilient communities shines brightly as a beacon of hope and change. The challenges of weak routine immunization, poor leadership and governance, poor coordination of disease outbreak and response, and non-performing primary healthcare centres are formidable but not insurmountable. Throughout this exploration, we have witnessed the resilience and determination of communities as they confront these challenges head-on.

Case Study 31: *Reviving Immunisation in the M Community: A Race Against Time.*

Introduction: The M community, nestled deep in the heart of a developing nation, was facing a looming threat due to weak routine immunisation. Childhood immunisation rates have steadily declined over the years, leading to outbreaks of vaccine-preventable diseases and putting children's health at risk.

Challenges:

1. Vaccine Hesitancy: A significant portion of the community was sceptical of vaccines, driven by misinformation and cultural beliefs.

2. Supply Chain Issues: Frequent stockouts of vaccines at the local health centre hindered regular immunisation services.

3. Limited Healthcare Workforce: The healthcare centre was understaffed, lacking trained personnel to administer vaccines.

Community Action: Realising the urgency of the situation, a group of concerned parents and community leaders came together. They organised awareness campaigns, engaging local influencers and elders to address vaccine hesitancy. They also collaborated with healthcare workers to ensure a consistent supply of vaccines and organised mobile immunisation clinics to reach remote areas of the community.

Results: Over time, the community's concerted efforts led to a significant increase in immunisation rates. The number of children receiving vaccines grew steadily, leading to a decline in vaccine-preventable diseases in the M community.

Lessons Learned: This case study underscores the vital role of community engagement and empowerment in overcoming challenges related to weak routine immunisation. It demonstrates that through collective action and education, communities can revitalise immunisation programs and protect the health of their children.

Case Study 32: *Transforming Governance for Health in the X Republic*

Introduction: The X Republic, a developing nation, had long grappled with poor leadership and governance in its healthcare system. Inefficient resource allocation, corruption, and lack of transparency have hindered the progress of public health initiatives.

Challenges:

1. Resource Mismanagement: Funds meant for healthcare were frequently misallocated, leading to the underfunding of critical health programs.

2. Corruption: Instances of corruption and embezzlement within the healthcare system eroded public trust and hampered effective service delivery.

3. Lack of Accountability: The absence of clear accountability structures allowed inefficiencies to persist unchecked.

Community Action: Citizens of the Republic of X, weary of subpar healthcare, joined forces to demand transparency and accountability. They organised public protests, collaborated with investigative journalists, and formed local watchdog groups to monitor healthcare spending.

Results: The pressure from the community and civil society led to a wave of anti-corruption reforms in the healthcare system. New leadership emerged, committed to transparency and accountability. Healthcare funds were reallocated effectively, and programs addressing critical public health issues were revitalised.

Lessons Learned: This case study highlights the transformative power of community advocacy and the importance of holding leaders and institutions accountable. Through collective action, communities can drive change and help overcome barriers imposed by poor leadership and governance.

Case Study 33: *Unifying Response: Tackling the Cholera Outbreak in the Y Region*

Introduction: The Y region in a developing nation had a history of poor coordination during disease outbreaks. The recent cholera outbreak threatened the lives of thousands, exposing systemic flaws in the response.

Challenges:

1. *Lack of Communication:* Multiple agencies and organisations involved in the response had difficulty sharing crucial information.

2. *Resource Duplication:* Resources were duplicated, resulting in inefficient allocation during the outbreak.

3. *Delayed Response:* The lack of coordination led to delays in response efforts, causing the outbreak to spread.

Community Action: Community leaders, local health workers, and NGOs recognised the urgency of the situation. They initiated regular coordination meetings, established a centralised information-sharing platform, and coordinated resource allocation. They engaged community members in surveillance efforts to identify and isolate cases promptly.

Results: The improved coordination led to a more effective response. Cholera cases were identified and treated swiftly, while public health campaigns educated the community about preventive measures. The outbreak was controlled, and the Uvilon region began developing a coordinated response plan for future health crises.

Lessons Learned: This case study emphasises the importance of local coordination and the central role that resilient communities can play in enhancing the response to disease outbreaks. It shows that by addressing communication and resource allocation issues, communities can minimise the impact of health crises.

Case Study 34: *Community-Led Healthcare: Rejuvenating Primary Care in the M District*

Introduction: In the M district of a developing nation, underperforming primary healthcare centres have resulted in limited access to healthcare services, particularly in rural areas.

Challenges:

1. ***Lack of Infrastructure:*** Primary healthcare centres were understaffed and lacked essential medical equipment.

2. ***Geographic Disparities:*** Rural communities face long distances to access healthcare, discouraging regular visits.

3. ***Inadequate Healthcare Workforce:*** The shortage of trained healthcare professionals limited the quality of care.

Community Action: Frustrated by these challenges, community members in M took matters into their own hands. They organized community health workers, established mobile clinics, and engaged in fundraising efforts to improve healthcare infrastructure. Local leaders advocated for government support to rejuvenate primary healthcare centres.

Results: The community-led healthcare initiatives in M significantly improved healthcare access. Mobile clinics ensured that even remote areas received medical attention. The M district government responded by investing in healthcare infrastructure and increasing the workforce.

Lessons Learned: This case study highlights the potential for community-driven initiatives to bridge gaps in healthcare access, even in resource-constrained settings. It demonstrates that resilient communities can play a pivotal role in advocating for and rejuvenating primary healthcare centres, ultimately improving healthcare services for all.

CONCLUSION

Resilient communities serve as pivotal agents of change in navigating public health challenges within developing nations. Through their empowerment, advocacy, collaboration, and innovative approaches, they contribute significantly to improving health outcomes, promoting health equity, and enhancing community well-being. Despite facing formidable obstacles, resilient communities offer hope and inspiration for creating healthier and more resilient societies, demonstrating the transformative potential of local-level action and community-driven initiatives.

REFERENCES

[1] WHO. Immunization. World Health Organization, 2021. Available from: https://www.who.int/health-topics/immunization

[2] Orenstein WA, Ahmed R. Simply put: Vaccination saves lives. Proc Natl Acad Sci USA 2017; 114(16): 4031-3.
[http://dx.doi.org/10.1073/pnas.1704507114] [PMID: 28396427]

[3] Kickbusch, I., & Gleicher, D. Governance for health in the 21st century. World Health Organization 2012. Available from: https://iris.who.int/handle/10665/326429

[4] Bossert TJ, Beauvais JC. Decentralization of health systems in Ghana, Zambia, Uganda and the Philippines: a comparative analysis of decision space. Health Policy Plan 2002; 17(1): 14-31.
[http://dx.doi.org/10.1093/heapol/17.1.14] [PMID: 11861583]

[5] WHO. International Health Regulations Third Edition. World Health Organization, 2017. Available from: https://www.who.int/publications/i/item/9789241580496

[6] Heymann DL, Rodier GR. Hot spots in a wired world: WHO surveillance of emerging and re-emerging infectious diseases. Lancet Infect Dis 2001; 1(5): 345-53.
[http://dx.doi.org/10.1016/S1473-3099(01)00148-7] [PMID: 11871807]

[7] Osewe PL. Options for financing pandemic preparedness. Bull World Health Organ 2017; 95(12): 794-794A.
[http://dx.doi.org/10.2471/BLT.17.199695] [PMID: 29200516]

[8] WHO. The World Health Report 2008: Primary Health Care - Now More Than Ever. World Health Organization, 2008. Available from: https://www.who.int/director-general/speeches/detail/primar--health-care---now-more-than-ever

[9] Kruk ME, Ling EJ, Bitton A, *et al.* Building resilient health systems: a proposal for a resilience index. BMJ 2017; 357: j2323.
[http://dx.doi.org/10.1136/bmj.j2323] [PMID: 28536191]

[10]   WHO. Primary Health Care Programme in the WHO African Region from Alma-Ata to Ouagadougou and beyond, 2018. Available from: https://www.who.int/docs/default-source/primary-health-c-re-conference/phc-regional-report-africa.pdf?sfvrsn=73f1301f_2

[11]   Colten, C. E., Kates, R. W., and Laska, S. B. Community Resilience: Lessons from New Orleans and Hurricane Katrina. CARRI Report, 2008; 3. Available from: https://www.rwkates.org/pdfs/a2008.03.pdf

[12]   Cutter SL, Barnes L, Berry M, *et al.* A place-based model for understanding community resilience to natural disasters. Glob Environ Change 2008; 18(4): 598-606.
[http://dx.doi.org/10.1016/j.gloenvcha.2008.07.013]

[13]   Norris FH, Stevens SP, Pfefferbaum B, Wyche KF, Pfefferbaum RL. Community resilience as a metaphor, theory, set of capacities, and strategy for disaster readiness. Am J Community Psychol 2008; 41(1-2): 127-50.
[http://dx.doi.org/10.1007/s10464-007-9156-6] [PMID: 18157631]

CHAPTER 18

Conclusion

Abstract: Chapter 18 serves as the conclusion to the book, "Resilient Communities: Navigating Public Health Challenges in Developing Nations." It provides a comprehensive summary of key insights and takeaways from the preceding chapters, highlighting the critical role of resilient communities in addressing public health challenges. The chapter concludes with a call to action for building resilient communities and improving public health in developing nations through collaboration, investment, empowerment, innovation, and sustainable development approaches.

Keywords: Call to action, Collaboration, Developing nations, Empowerment, Investment, Innovation, Public health challenges, Resilient communities, Summary, Sustainable development.

INTRODUCTION

Chapter 18 offers a synthesis of the diverse themes explored throughout the book, emphasizing the importance of resilient communities in tackling public health challenges in developing nations. It reflects on key insights, strategies, and interventions discussed in preceding chapters, underscoring the interconnectedness of health, development, and community well-being. The chapter sets the stage for a call to action, urging stakeholders to collectively work towards building resilient communities and shaping a healthier future.

Summary of Key Insights and Takeaways

Throughout this book, we have explored the critical role of resilient communities in navigating public health challenges in developing nations. From understanding the public health challenges specific to these regions to exploring strategies and interventions, each chapter has provided valuable insights into building a healthier and more sustainable future. Here are some key takeaways from our journey:

1. Resilient Communities: Resilience is the cornerstone of effective public health responses in developing nations. Empowering communities to withstand and recover from health challenges is essential for achieving better health outcomes.

2. Addressing Communicable Diseases: Preventing and controlling infectious diseases requires a multi-pronged approach, including vaccination campaigns, disease surveillance, and effective outbreak management.

3. Non-Communicable Diseases and Lifestyle Interventions: Tackling non-communicable diseases necessitates promoting healthy behaviors, ensuring access to healthcare, and addressing socio-economic factors influencing public health.

4. Maternal and Child Health: Enhancing maternal care, childhood immunization, and effective management of common childhood illnesses are fundamental to improving maternal and child health outcomes.

5. Healthcare Infrastructure and Access: Strengthening healthcare facilities, overcoming access barriers, and embracing telemedicine and innovative healthcare models can improve healthcare access and delivery.

6. Water, Sanitation, and Hygiene (WASH) Interventions: Access to clean water and sanitation is vital for disease prevention and community well-being, making WASH interventions crucial for public health.

7. Nutrition and Food Security: Addressing malnutrition and food insecurity requires sustainable agriculture, community food initiatives, and empowering communities to improve nutrition.

8. Mental Health and Psychosocial Support: Recognizing mental health challenges and integrating psychosocial support into public health programs are essential for overall community well-being.

9. Disaster Preparedness and Resilience: Building community resilience and learning from past disaster responses enhance preparedness and response to emergencies and natural disasters.

10. Empowering Women and Girls in Public Health: Advancing gender equity, promoting women's health, and empowering girls through education and health initiatives lead to stronger and more resilient communities.

11. Technology and Innovation in Public Health: Harnessing technology, mHealth, eHealth initiatives, and digital tools for data collection and analysis drive transformative improvements in public health practices.

12. Sustainable Development and Resilient Health Futures: Integrating public health into sustainable development goals, fostering community resilience, and shaping a healthier future are vital for building resilient health systems.

Call to Action for Building Resilient Communities and Improving Public Health in Developing Nations

As we conclude this book, it is clear that the path to resilient communities and improved public health in developing nations requires collective efforts and committed action. Here's a call to action for all stakeholders involved in shaping public health:

1. Collaboration and Partnerships: Governments, international organizations, non-governmental organizations, communities, and the private sector must collaborate and form strong partnerships to address complex public health challenges together.

2. Investment in Health Systems: Investing in robust and inclusive health systems is essential for building resilience and ensuring equitable access to quality healthcare for all.

3. Empowerment and Inclusivity: Empowering communities, especially women and girls, through education, health initiatives, and meaningful participation in decision-making processes fosters ownership and inclusivity in public health interventions.

4. Innovation and Technology: Embracing innovation and technology can revolutionize public health practices, enhance data collection and analysis, and bridge gaps in healthcare access.

5. Sustainable Development Approach: Integrating public health into sustainable development goals promotes a holistic approach to addressing health challenges while considering social, economic, and environmental dimensions.

6. Disaster Preparedness and Response: Strengthening disaster preparedness and response capacities ensures timely and effective interventions during emergencies.

7. Health Equity and Social Justice: Addressing health inequalities and disparities is essential for building resilient communities and achieving health equity.

8. Education and Awareness: Promoting health education and awareness campaigns empowers individuals to take charge of their health and well-being.

In the journey through the preceding chapters, "Resilient Communities: Navigating Public Health Challenges in Developing Nations" has explored the intricate tapestry of challenges and opportunities that define the public health landscape in developing nations. From the rise of non-communicable diseases to maternal and child health, healthcare infrastructure, disaster preparedness, and beyond, the book has endeavored to provide a comprehensive understanding of how resilient communities can emerge from the intersections of health, development, and human well-being.

The Intersection of Health and Development: At the heart of this exploration lies the recognition that health and development are inseparable companions on the path to progress. The symbiotic relationship between public health and sustainable development underscores that a nation's vitality depends on the well-being of its citizens. Through this interplay, the book has illuminated how investing in health not only safeguards communities against disease but also fortifies their capacity to withstand adversity and contribute to broader societal growth.

Themes of Resilience and Empowerment: The resounding theme throughout these chapters is resilience—the capacity of communities to adapt, overcome challenges, and thrive in the face of adversity. The book has underscored that resilience is not just an outcome; it is a mindset, a set of values, and a collective commitment to building a brighter future. Resilience hinges on empowerment—empowering individuals, families, and communities with knowledge, skills, and resources to take charge of their health and well-being.

Foundations for a Healthier Future: As the chapters unfolded, it became evident that public health challenges cannot be addressed in isolation. Whether it's the integration of public health into sustainable development goals or the pursuit of gender equity, the book has elucidated the critical role of partnerships, collaboration, and holistic approaches in shaping a healthier future. The discussions on technology, innovation, and capacity building have revealed the transformative potential of collective action and innovation in advancing public health.

The Way Forward: In the final analysis, "Resilient Communities: Navigating Public Health Challenges in Developing Nations" is not just a collection of chapters; it is a call to action. It beckons policymakers, healthcare professionals, community leaders, and citizens to come together and forge a path that leads to resilient, equitable, and sustainable communities. It emphasizes that while challenges may be formidable, the potential for positive change is equally immense.

Building resilient communities and improving public health in developing nations is not an insurmountable task. It requires a collective commitment to addressing health challenges, fostering community empowerment, and investing in sustainable health systems. By embracing innovation, inclusivity, and a sustainable development approach, we can create a future where communities thrive, public health is safeguarded, and no one is left behind in the pursuit of a healthier and more resilient world. Together, let us embark on this journey towards building resilient communities and shaping a brighter future for all. As we conclude this exploration of resilient communities, it's clear that the journey ahead is multifaceted and demanding. The path to healthier, more resilient communities requires a steadfast commitment to improving healthcare infrastructure, empowering women and girls, addressing malnutrition, harnessing technology, and much more. It necessitates cross-sectoral collaboration, innovative solutions, and a shared vision of progress.

"Resilient Communities: Navigating Public Health Challenges in Developing Nations" has sought to inspire change-makers, spark conversations, and offer a compass for navigating the complex landscape of public health. The journey doesn't end here; it evolves as we collectively strive to transform challenges into opportunities, adversities into triumphs, and setbacks into springboards for progress.

Sustainable development goals have provided a vision for resilient health futures in developing nations, emphasizing integrating public health into long-term resilience efforts. The stories in this book serve as a testament to the transformative potential of local-level action, community-driven initiatives, and the unyielding spirit of communities in the face of adversity.

This book is not merely a compilation of knowledge but an invitation to action. It is a call to embrace the resilience within us all and recognize that the most potent solutions emerge when we work together as a global community united in purpose and compassion. May the book serve as a reminder that each action, no matter how small, contributes to the grand tapestry of resilient communities - a tapestry woven with dedication, innovation, and the unwavering belief in the potential for a healthier, more equitable future.

GLOSSARY

In this comprehensive glossary, we provide key terms and their definitions that have been introduced and discussed throughout this handbook. The glossary provides definitions for key terms and concepts discussed throughout the book, helping readers to better understand the context and significance of the topics addressed.

Resilient Communities: Communities that demonstrate the ability to adapt, withstand, and recover from adversity, including public health challenges, through collective action, resourcefulness, and empowerment.

Public Health Challenges: Various obstacles and issues that affect the health and well-being of populations, including infectious diseases, inadequate healthcare infrastructure, poor sanitation, malnutrition, and limited access to healthcare services.

Developing Nations: Countries or regions characterized by lower levels of economic development often face challenges such as poverty, limited access to healthcare, inadequate infrastructure, and socio-economic disparities.

Health Equity: The principle of ensuring that all individuals have the opportunity to attain their highest level of health, regardless of socio-economic status, geographic location, or other factors that may contribute to disparities in health outcomes.

Maternal and Child Health: The health and well-being of mothers and children, including prenatal care, childbirth, postnatal care, and childhood health interventions aimed at reducing maternal and child mortality and morbidity.

Non-Communicable Diseases (NCDs): Chronic diseases that are not passed from person to person, including conditions such as cardiovascular diseases, cancer, diabetes, and chronic respiratory diseases.

Communicable Diseases: Illnesses caused by infectious agents or pathogens that can be transmitted from person to person, including bacteria, viruses, parasites, and fungi.

Healthcare Infrastructure: The physical and organizational structures that support the delivery of healthcare services, including hospitals, clinics, laboratories, medical equipment, and health information systems.

WASH Interventions: Interventions aimed at improving access to clean water, sanitation, and hygiene practices to prevent waterborne diseases and promote community well-being.

Nutrition and Food Security: Efforts to ensure that individuals and communities have access to an adequate and nutritious diet, addressing issues such as food insecurity, malnutrition, and micronutrient deficiencies.

Mental Health: The psychological and emotional well-being of individuals and communities, including efforts to promote mental wellness, prevent mental disorders, and provide support and treatment for those experiencing mental health challenges.

Disaster Preparedness and Response: Measures taken to mitigate the impact of disasters, including natural disasters such as earthquakes, floods, and hurricanes, as well as human-made disasters such as conflicts and industrial accidents.

Empowerment: The process of enabling individuals and communities to take control of their own lives, make informed decisions, and advocate for their rights and interests.

Gender Equity: The principle of ensuring fairness and equality between men and women, including equal access to opportunities, resources, and rights in all aspects of life, including healthcare, education, and employment.

Sustainable Development: Development that meets the needs of the present without compromising the ability of future generations to meet their own needs, integrating social, economic, and environmental considerations.

Innovation and Technology: The use of new ideas, methods, and technologies to address public health challenges, improve healthcare delivery, and enhance data collection, analysis, and communication.

Collaboration and Partnerships: Cooperative efforts between governments, non-governmental organizations, communities, and other stakeholders to address complex public health challenges through shared resources, expertise, and responsibilities.

Health Systems Strengthening: Efforts to improve the capacity, efficiency, and effectiveness of health systems, including investments in infrastructure, workforce development, service delivery, and governance.

Community Engagement: Involving community members in decision-making processes, program planning, implementation, and evaluation to ensure that interventions are culturally appropriate, sustainable, and responsive to local needs.

Capacity Building: Enhancing the knowledge, skills, and resources of individuals and organizations to improve their ability to address public health challenges, including training, education, mentorship, and organizational development initiatives.

SUBJECT INDEX

www.ingramcontent.com/pod-product-compliance
Lightning Source LLC
Chambersburg PA
CBHW041659210326

41598CB00007B/459